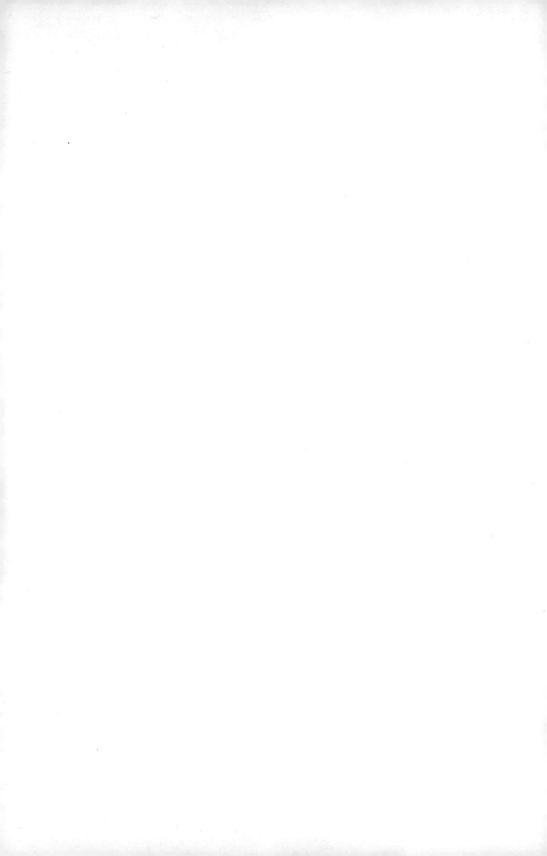

CONDOM NATION

CONDOM NATION

*The U.S. Government's
Sex Education Campaign from
World War I to the Internet*

Alexandra M. Lord

The Johns Hopkins University Press
Baltimore

© 2010 The Johns Hopkins University Press
All rights reserved. Published 2010
Printed in the United States of America on acid-free paper
9 8 7 6 5 4 3 2 1

The Johns Hopkins University Press
2715 North Charles Street
Baltimore, Maryland 21218-4363
www.press.jhu.edu

Library of Congress Cataloging-in-Publication Data
Lord, Alexandra M.
    Condom nation : the U.S. government's sex education campaign
from World War I to the Internet / Alexandra M. Lord.
        p. cm.
    Includes bibliographical references and index.
    ISBN-13: 978-0-8018-9380-3 (hardcover : alk. paper)
    ISBN-10: 0-8018-9380-1 (hardcover : alk. paper)
    I. Title.
    [DNLM: 1. United States. Public Health Service. 2. Sex
Education—history—United States. 3. Contraception—United
States. 4. Government Programs—history—United States. 5. History,
20th Century—United States. 6. Sexually Transmitted Diseases—
prevention & control—United States. 7. United States Government
Agencies—history—United States. HQ 31 L866c 2009]
    HQ31.L817 2009
    613.9071′073—dc22   2009006038

A catalog record for this book is available from the British Library.

Special discounts are available for bulk purchases of this book.
For more information, please contact Special Sales at 410-516-6936
or specialsales@press.jhu.edu.

The Johns Hopkins University Press uses environmentally friendly
book materials, including recycled text paper that is composed of at
least 30 percent post-consumer waste, whenever possible. All of our
book papers are acid-free, and our jackets and covers are printed on
paper with recycled content.

For Ben,

die wege mit dir—
sie hinterlassen spuren
in meinem herzen

CONTENTS

ACKNOWLEDGMENTS

Writing a book is never a solitary project. I have benefited tremendously from the suggestions and knowledge of many people.

Within the Office of the Public Health Service Historian and the Department of Health and Human Services, Victoria Harden, Sheena Morrison, John Parascandola, John Swann, Lindsey Hobbs, Cindy Lachin, and Suzanne Junod all provided support and assistance. John Parascandola generously shared his work with me, commenting as well on my own work. John Swann, Sheena Morrison, and Lindsey Hobbs in particular shared my amusement about the history of sex education, and our many discussions about this topic made writing this book a great deal of fun.

At the National Archives, Marjorie Ciarlante was extremely helpful in steering me toward the documents and materials I needed. Stephen Greenberg at the National Library of Medicine provided me with similar assistance, as did David Klaassen at the Kautz Family YMCA Archives and Social Welfare History (ASHA) Archives at the University of Minnesota. Versions of chapter 2 appeared previously as "Models of Masculinity: Sex Education, the YMCA and the United States Public Health Service," *Journal of the History of Medicine and Allied Sciences*, vol. 58, no. 2 (2003), and "Naturally Clean and Wholesome: Women, Sex Education and the United States Public Heath Service, 1918–1928," *Social History of Medicine*, vol. 17, no. 3 (2004). An overview of broader beliefs about sex education also appeared in " 'Learning the Washington Way': The United States Public Health Service and the Problem of Sex Education, 1919–1996," *Occasional Papers of the Society of History in the Federal Government* (2004). I have presented papers about the history of sex education at many conferences (the American Public Health Association, the Organization of American Historians, the American Association for the History of Medicine, the History of Science Society, the Society for History in the Federal Government, and the Washington Society for the History of Medicine), and I have given talks about sex education at George Washington University, the National Library of

Medicine, Pennsylvania State University, York, and Clarkson University. Audience members as well as the editors and reviewers of my earlier articles provided excellent comments and suggestions, many of which are incorporated here.

At the Johns Hopkins University Press, Jacqueline Wehmueller has been everything an editor can and should be. Her patience as this project unfolded was central to ensuring its completion. I also appreciate the copy-editing work of Mary Yates and the comments of an anonymous reviewer.

Over the past seven years I have benefited tremendously from my friendships with historians in and outside the academy. David Cantor, Judy Chelnick, Liz Fee, Caroline Hannaway, Andrew Harris, Alan Kraut, Sarah Leavitt, Mike Lynn, Michelle McClellan, Marla Miller, Mike Sappol, Leo Slater, Phil Teigen, and Anne Whisnant have all encouraged me to think broadly about why history really does matter. More generally, the communities of Beyond Academe and Wrk4Us have taught me to think about why scholars should try to reach a wide audience.

More recently, the support of my colleagues has been instrumental in helping me to complete this project. I am especially grateful to Jamie Jacobs, Linda McClelland, Erika Martin Seibert, and Bob Sutton, all of whom shared their thoughts on writing with me. Kate Richards and Alexis Abernathy very kindly provided me with their considerable expertise on photography. Paul Loether, my boss, was also very supportive of this project.

In Washington, D.C., Ray and Adele Natter, Klaus Decker, Wayne Thomas, and Lars Reihoff have been wonderful friends, and I have appreciated their interest in this project as it progressed. Ray and Adele's stories about Ray's working a nine-to-five job while writing legal textbooks gave me the impetus I needed to write on the weekend and in the evening. Lars also patiently endured my wild enthusiasm for things Danish and kindly provided me with a Danish perspective on public health, Danish society, and its many differences from American society. *Tak*, Lars.

Even as I doubted my ability to complete this book, my family never wavered in their belief that I could do this. Adam Apt, Sara Lord, Rob Storch, Charlotte and Hannah Storch, Christopher Lord, Cynthia Ogden, Benjamin and Katya Ogden-Lord, Victoria Lord, Mark Eckenwiler, Nicholas and Caleb Eckenwiler, Barbara and Tom Roberts, and Eleanor Kaplan have all expressed complete and utter confidence that I would do this, and I am thankful for their belief in me.

Laura Ettinger and I met as undergraduates at Vassar College, where she raised the question of whether majoring in history was "a good idea." Since our first meeting, Laura has been a wonderful friend and colleague. Our very long and still ongoing conversation about why it is a "good idea" to study history has deeply influenced this book. Her multiple invitations to speak to her under-graduate students and colleagues at Clarkson University about the history of sex education provided me with wonderful opportunities to think broadly about the history of the subject. Laura also went above and beyond the limits of friendship by reading the entire book, in its many different forms, offering com-ments and suggestions. She was always available when I called to ask "just one more thing."

Long before college, my parents, Athena and Victor Lord, introduced me to the joys of libraries and reading. I am more grateful to them than they will ever know for teaching me to "look it up!" Since my father's premature death, my mother has been wonderful, sharing my interest in and passion for history and encouraging me in both my career and my writing. A prize-winning children's author, she has taught me a great deal about good writing, and on the rare oc-casions when she has not directly edited my work, she has shaped it through her general comments and suggestions. This book owes a great deal to her teach-ings. *Ευχαριστώ μητέρα.*

Every medical historian should have ready access to a health policy analyst and attorney. I have been especially fortunate in that I married one. Benjamin L. Apt, my husband, helped me to understand how the legislative process works and how health policies are enforced at the federal, state, and local levels. Ben's constant questioning and passion for history has made me a better historian; it has also greatly enhanced my life. Finally, while I recommend marrying a health policy analyst, I'd also recommend marrying the son of a copy-editor. Ben proved that copy-editing is genetic by carefully editing my work and ensuring that my writing was clear. *Ich liebe dich*, Ben.

A WORD ON TERMINOLOGY

Over the past hundred years as our views of sex education, sexually transmitted diseases, and out-of-wedlock births have changed, the terminology used to describe these concepts has also shifted. As a historian I prefer to use the terminology that was in vogue during the period under study. As a result, the first part of this book discusses *venereal diseases, illegitimate births,* and the idea of *continence,* while the second part focuses on *sexually transmitted diseases, unwanted pregnancies* and *out-of-wedlock births,* and the concept of *abstinence.*

Similar problems emerge when discussing various organizations and federal agencies whose names have changed over the past hundred years. The Communicable Disease Center (later renamed the Centers for Disease Control and Prevention) and the American Social Hygiene Association (later renamed the American Social Health Association) wisely retained their abbreviations when they renamed themselves, but not every organization was so far-sighted. I try whenever possible to use common abbreviations throughout the book, but I also need, on occasion, to refer to these organizations by their full name. In those instances I always use the name that was commonly used at that time. Similarly, I use the historical names for other organizations whose names have changed over time.

CONDOM NATION

CHAPTER ONE

IN BED WITH THE FED

If young people of both sexes can be impressed with the dignity and true significance of sex, sordid experiences will tend to lessen and thus decrease the possible exposure to venereal disease.

SURGEON GENERAL HUGH S. CUMMING, 1926

If we had good education of children by their parents, if that education was reinforced in schools with moral, responsible sex education, and that was also reinforced in the churches, I believe we could reach the end result that I am looking for: we could raise the next generation of adolescents to be abstinent until monogamous.

SURGEON GENERAL C. EVERETT KOOP, 1988

I t was, the headlines screamed, a "case of too much candor." On December 1, 1994, World AIDS Day, Surgeon General Joycelyn Elders publicly announced that masturbation "is part of human sexuality and it's a part of something that perhaps should be taught."[1] Within the week Elders' excessive candor had resulted in her being fired. For reporters, it was a dream story—the culture wars writ large in the fate of one individual, an African-American pediatrician from a small town in Arkansas who had risen to become surgeon general.

Elders had come to Washington, D.C., in 1993 as a relentless crusader for sex education. Vilified as the "condom queen" by her opponents, she kept an arrangement of faux flowers on her desk. Fashioned from condom wrappers, they served to remind her of her primary goals: reducing teen pregnancy and arresting the spread of sexually transmitted diseases.[2] But in the year and a half after her confirmation she had failed to make much progress toward achieving either of these goals. She had, however, succeeded in becoming a lightning rod for the Far Right. By December of 1994 the attacks had become so vitriolic that even her supporters, such as the beleaguered president, Bill Clinton, had been forced to distance themselves from her. In her remarks on World AIDS Day her opponents found and gleefully exploited her Achilles heel: her tendency to speak bluntly and off-script about sex education. For public health experts and news watchers, Elders' fall was not a surprise. The surprise had been her ability to hold on to power for so long.

Elders' fall and the storm of controversy that exploded over her comments about sex education were nothing new. Long before she spoke about the need for both more openness about masturbation and more innovative approaches to sex education, her predecessors, Surgeons General Rupert Blue, Hugh S. Cumming, Thomas Parran, William Stewart, Jesse Steinfeld, C. Everett Koop, and Antonia Novello had struggled to provide the American public with information about sexually transmitted diseases and human sexuality, usually in the face of disapproving administrations and private organizations. And years after her firing, her successors, David Satcher and Richard Carmona, would struggle with the same issues.

Throughout the twentieth century, battles over sex education have been at the center of broader discussions about the nation's health. Today we speak about the AIDS crisis that plagues our inner cities and is creeping into rural America. We speak firmly about the need to arrest this epidemic by any means possible. Few of us are aware, however, that a hundred years ago Americans made similar pronouncements lamenting the spread of venereal disease within the nation's cities and rural areas and calling for the government to intervene and arrest the epidemic. Then as now, sex education has been widely regarded as a crucial tool in fighting these epidemics. Then as now, the federal government has been seen as the best mechanism to provide this education. But sex education has proved to be an explosive catalyst, causing public health experts to lose their jobs and some Americans to rail against the federal government's encroachment into the most private aspects of our daily lives. These reactions to federally funded sex education programs have reflected Americans' uneasiness with sexual behavior as well as their ambivalence toward the power of the federal government.[3]

Since the nation's inception, governments at the local, state, and federal levels have advocated programs to promote Americans' health. In the early twentieth century the growth of interest groups such as the American Public Health Association, the rise of new professions, and the development of interconnected bureaucracies at the federal, state, and local levels all combined to give a new impetus to these programs.[4] Reflecting the goals of interest groups that were eager to protect Americans from the cradle to the grave, the federal government partnered with state and local governments as well as the medical and teaching professions to advocate the teaching of sex education. Funded primarily by federal grants to states, these sex education programs were cast as community initiatives, and as such they were extraordinarily popular. During the 1930s, as federal power and the federal bureaucracy expanded, sex education became centralized. The federal government took a more active role in promoting these initiatives and dictating the use of funding to promote them. When America went to war in 1941, all young men who were eligible for the draft received sex education directly from the government; at home, their sweethearts and sisters were treated to a barrage of similar programs. By the postwar era, the growth of federal agencies that promoted public health ensured that the federal government would continue to play an extremely active role in promoting sex education. Responses to sex education have never been uniform, but Americans generally viewed these programs in a positive light until the late 1960s and mid-1970s, when a general backlash against the federal government sparked a similar backlash against these programs. By the election of Ronald Reagan as president in 1981, a growing number of Americans were publicly—and loudly—questioning the role the federal government should play in promoting sex education. The advent of the AIDS crisis highlighted these tensions and revealed a series of deep divides in American society. As concerns over AIDS shifted in the 1990s, criticisms of government "meddling" in sex education intensified. Yet even as federally funded sex education programs came under attack, the federal government continued to play the major role in shaping, either directly or indirectly, the sex education available to most Americans.

The ensuing debates over sex education have often been portrayed as debates over the issue of medicine and morality. President Ronald Reagan tackled this issue directly when he insisted that sex education "can not be what some call 'value neutral.' After all," he asked, "when it comes to preventing AIDS, don't medicine and morality teach the same lessons?"[5] Reagan's question was a troubling one for public health experts. It lacked the nuanced understanding they have repeatedly demanded when teaching adolescents and even adults about sex. Medicine and morality are not, many sex educators would say, diametrically opposed—nor are they synonymous. Rather, they are two different and unrelated issues. Throughout the long history of American sex education programs, the desire to conflate these two issues or to set them up in opposition to one another has caused incalculable and often irreparable damage to both privately and federally funded sex education programs.

By structuring the debate over sex education as a debate over medicine and morality, opponents and even proponents of sex education have pushed sex educators into an either/or situation. Either one supports medical science or one supports morality. One cannot support both. This type of division enables each side of the sex education debate to characterize their detractors as opponents of morality or enemies of medical progress. Structuring the debate in these terms has mired sex education programs in broader ideological disputes. Nowhere has this controversy been more evident than in the long history of federally funded sex education programs.

The roots of the debates over sex education are more complex than simple arguments about medicine and morality would have us believe. These debates also reflect America's history of racial and religious prejudice as well as its very real social divisions. In the early twentieth century, sex education campaigns appealed to most Americans because syphilis and gonorrhea threatened everyone, regardless of class, race, religion, or geographic location. Throughout the twentieth century the government increasingly refined its programs, tailoring the message to meet the needs of specific groups. As sex education programs increasingly came to be associated with specific subsections of the population, such as homosexuals or urban and minority teens, these programs came under attack. These attacks reflected other criticisms of entitlement programs that were also seen as serving a subsection of the population. Religion continued, of course, to play a significant role in shaping these debates, but the attacks on sex education programs that emerged between the late 1960s and well into the 1980s often emanated from suburban and middle-class constituencies that were also critical of welfare and other programs associated with the New Deal and Johnson's Great Society.[6]

All of these disputes have resulted in a schizophrenic approach to sex education by the federal government over the last hundred years. More so than independently funded sex education campaigns, the government's sex education programs, conducted under the aegis of the Public Health Service, have been shaped by popular opinion—which has been swayed by the broader divisions in American society. Understanding the tensions between these divisions requires an in-depth understanding of the origins of federally funded sex education and the problems that have dogged these programs. Only when we understand how and why the government became involved in sex education, and the problems and successes that have marked the government's ninety-year campaign, can we begin to address the pressing questions that confront sex education programs today.

From Maritime to Public Health

From its founding, the American state has shaped the lives of its citizens in ways both obvious and hidden.[7] The active intervention of the state in protecting its citizens' health has been central to American history. Shaped by Enlightenment ideals that championed science, the nation's founders saw a strong link between the country's economic prosperity and the health and well-being of the its citizens. Because most goods were transported by water, Congress viewed seamen as playing a major role in contributing to the nation's prosperity. In 1798, Congress approved the creation of a fund designed for the "temporary relief and maintenance of sick or disabled seamen."[8] The Act mandated the deduction of 20 cents each month from the salaries of all American seamen; this money was used to fund the Marine Hospital Service, a federal institution that built and supervised a series of hospitals in the nation's port cities. American seamen who became ill away from home were entitled to care in any of these hospitals.

Although this network of hospitals was primarily concerned with protecting the health of sailors, it also slowed the spread of epidemics, an especially crucial task in an age when the understanding of epidemiology was rudimentary and there were few remedies for most diseases. Simply by isolating sick sailors from healthy citizens, the Act provided port cities with some protection against epidemics.

Paralleling the rise of other similar federal institutions, the hospitals created by the Marine Hospital Fund grew dramatically in number during the first half of the nineteenth century.[9] By midcentury, Marine Hospitals served sailors in ports from New Orleans to Boston. The Act was deemed a major success in its early years, but problems developed. The fund was originally intended to provide health care for the nation's workforce, but it also came to enrich unscrupulous politicians, physicians, and builders. By the time of the Civil War the Marine Hospital Service was openly charged with running hospitals for political rather than maritime or health needs. These charges were not entirely without basis. By the end of the Civil War, only eight of the Service's twenty-seven hospitals functioned according to their original purpose.

Facing mounting criticism, the Treasury Department, which oversaw the Marine Hospital Service, initiated a study of the fund and its network of hospitals in 1869. The Service's detractors assumed that the study would recommend the closure of the hospitals, but reflecting a broader trend toward the expansion of government services, it called instead for the Service to continue, although

with several fundamental changes. The most important of these recommendations called for the creation of a "Supervising Surgeon of the Marine Hospital."
The "supervising surgeon" would oversee the Fund and ensure that the hospitals were properly staffed and efficiently run. John Maynard Woodworth, the
first supervising surgeon, initiated a radical overhaul of the existing system.
Over the course of the next twenty years, Woodworth and his two immediate
successors transformed the Service into a dynamic and highly professionalized
service that directly cared for all Americans, not simply merchant marines.

Under Woodworth's reforms, physicians who wanted to serve in the Marine
Hospital Service were required to pass a medical examination. At a time when
the nation's civil servants were awarded their jobs on the basis of whom they
knew, not what they knew, the Marine Hospital Service broke the mold by requiring its employees to demonstrate competence in their field. The require-
ments imposed by the Marine Hospital Service were also unusual within the
broader field of medicine, as nineteenth-century American physicians did not
need to attend medical school or pass licensing exams before setting up a practice. This lax approach to medical regulation meant not only that Woodworth's
reforms created the nation's most professionalized cadre of physicians but also
that many of the nation's best physicians, eager to work with their peers, were
drawn to the Service. Woodworth then put these physicians in uniform using a
cache of old Civil War uniforms, imposing upon them a culture of military obe-
dience, regimentation, and rigor. Doctors appointed to "general service" within
the Marine Hospital Service were mobile; they traveled around the nation to
confront health crises as they emerged.

In 1873 Woodworth adopted a new title, supervising surgeon general, and,
throughout the 1870s and 1880s he and succeeding surgeons general pushed
against the boundaries that limited the Marine Hospital Service. This push
reflected two growing trends in America: the growth of federal (as opposed to
local or state) power, and the emergence of public health as a highly professionalized and scientific field of inquiry.

The expansion of the Marine Hospital Service's powers to impose and enforce quarantines was typical of both of these trends. As one of the oldest methods of preventing the spread of disease, quarantines had been used by Western
governments to prevent the spread of disease since at least the Middle Ages. Because the Marine Hospital Service was intimately involved with the care of merchant marines, the control of quarantine and the regulation of the nation's ports
was a natural outgrowth of the Service's overall mission. Through quarantine

duties and the imposition of disease prevention tactics at the nation's ports the Service became involved in broader issues related to the nation's health overall.

During the late nineteenth century the Service gradually took on a range of public health activities including sanitation, vaccination, and the prevention of infectious diseases within all of the nation's growing cities, not simply its ports. By the turn of the century the Marine Hospital Service ensured that tenement dwellers had access to clean and safe water, that rural farmers were building privies that did not endanger their users, and that outbreaks of contagious and potentially fatal diseases such as bubonic plague were contained. Americans overwhelmingly remained unaware of the Service, but its officers had quietly and radically worked to make their lives safer, healthier, and longer.

Marine Hospital Service employees were also at the forefront of a broader social change. Beginning in the late nineteenth century, empirically based medicine—or scientific medicine—began to dominate the practice of American medicine. By the 1880s a growing number of scientists and physicians had come to believe that disease was spread by minute pathogenic organisms, or germs. This new theory sparked what is often referred to as the bacteriological revolution, which radically transformed the practice of medicine. While late-nineteenth- and early-twentieth-century physicians did not always understand which bacillus caused which disease, they were finally able to understand how diseases spread and how they could be contained.[10]

By the 1880s, germ theory had begun to influence public health initiatives and policies. Following this development, in 1887 the Marine Hospital Service created a bacteriological laboratory to diagnose and fight disease. The creation of the Hygienic Laboratory—the forerunner of the National Institutes of Health—presaged a new approach in the fight to control communicable diseases. Public health experts and employees of the Marine Hospital Service were now able to identify diseases through laboratory analysis and to move to arrest an epidemic in its earliest stages. Residents of Washington, D.C., including many congressional legislators, witnessed and directly benefitted from this expansion in the Service's abilities to control disease when a 1906 epidemic of typhoid threatened the nation's capital. Called in to find the source of the epidemic, the Service's officers undertook a massive epidemiological study. Over the course of several months they interviewed many of the city's residents and assessed the city's water supply, tracing it as it crossed multiple state boundaries. They also initiated an in-depth examination of the city's new water filtration plant. Finally, officers scrutinized the city's milk by testing cows in the surrounding rural districts of Maryland and Virginia and by investigating the city's dairies and creameries, even its ice cream makers. By the time the Service's officers had located the source of the epidemic—tainted milk—the nation's legislators had recognized the essential role the Service played, and they were willing to provide support in the form of a healthy budget.[11] The Service was now poised to take on more aggressive tactics to fight communicable diseases, a category that included sexually transmitted diseases such as syphilis and gonorrhea.

Even before the Marine Hospital Service had demonstrated the scale of its capabilities by resolving Washington's typhoid epidemic, congressional legislators were aware that the Service cared for the health of all American citizens, not just its sailors. In 1902, Congress had authorized that the Marine Hospital Service be officially renamed the Public Health and Marine Hospital Service. Ten years later, in 1912, the name was shortened to the Public Health Service (PHS), a name that reflected the mission the Service had already been fulfilling for over a hundred years.

Between 1880 and 1924, as PHS physicians examined twenty million immigrants at Ellis Island, Angel Island, and other quarantine stations, the PHS began to track and assess epidemics on a global scale. Domestic concerns continued to dominate, however, and in 1930 the roster of patients under the care of the Service expanded to include federal prisoners. That same year the Hygienic Laboratory was transformed into the National Institute of Health (later renamed the National Institutes of Health) and relocated to Bethesda, Maryland, where it would become a colossus in the field of medical research, including research into the causes and potential cures for new diseases such as AIDS.

It was during the 1930s that the Service would embark on its most controversial project. The Tuskegee Syphilis Experiment began as a study of untreated syphilis in African-American men. The study's origins stemmed as much from the mistaken belief that African-American men were more sexually promiscuous than their white counterparts as it did from a desire to understand the ravages of untreated syphilis. In short, the study reflected the beliefs of a racially segregated society and a racially segregated institution, the Public Health Service. None of the men who were subjected to this experiment gave their informed consent to participate. From the 1930s well into the early 1970s, these men were misled as to the purpose of the study and the state of their own health. The federal government also failed to provide these patients with adequate treatment for syphilis during the 1930s. Worse yet, after penicillin became the drug of choice for treating syphilis in the 1940s, the PHS failed to offer it to these men. The Tuskegee Syphilis Experiment was not revealed until 1972. That year, in the wake of congressional hearings, scientific researchers in and outside of the PHS became aware of the unchecked dangers inherent in unregulated medical research on human subjects.[12]

The Tuskegee Syphilis Experiment developed alongside a more comprehensive PHS-sponsored program designed to combat malaria. Beginning in the late 1930s the program for Malaria Control in War Areas (MCWA) sought to arrest and reverse the spread of malaria throughout the nation. Following World War II the MCWA became the Communicable Disease Center (CDC) and took on a broader mission: to prevent the spread of all infectious diseases within the United States. In the 1980s the CDC would discover and track the emergence of a new infectious disease, AIDS. This new, broader mission led the Centers for Disease Control and Prevention, as the agency was renamed, to take on a starring role in films ranging from *The Band Played On* to *Outbreak*. The agency also played guest roles on television shows ranging from *ER* to *House* and *Law and Order*.[13] Greater visibility led, in turn, to a growth in the CDC's power to initiate and effect change in how epidemics were tracked.

The aftermath of World War II also saw a massive reorganization throughout the federal government. In 1953 a new executive agency dedicated to public health, the Department of Health, Education, and Welfare (HEW), replaced the Federal Security Agency, the former home of the Public Health Service. Within this new department the PHS assumed a dominant role, taking on responsibility for the Indian Health Service (IHS) and the Food and Drug Administration (FDA).

As the tasks assigned to the Public Health Service grew in number, so too did its employees. Dentists, pharmacists, engineers, chemists, social workers, veterinarians, biologists, and nurses all entered the ranks of the Commissioned Corps, the uniformed branch of the PHS, during the first half of the twentieth century. Civilian employees in clerical and support positions also increased. To some degree the growth of the PHS reflected the overall expansion of government that occurred during the 1930s, 1940s, and 1950s, but it also reflected an increasing public confidence in the ability of science to conquer and control diseases.

While Europeans and Americans shared this confidence in science, American approaches to public health differed from their European counterparts. Since the early nineteenth century, nations with highly centralized governments, such as Sweden, have maintained a comprehensive control over their public health initiatives.[14] But in the United States, where the nation's founders

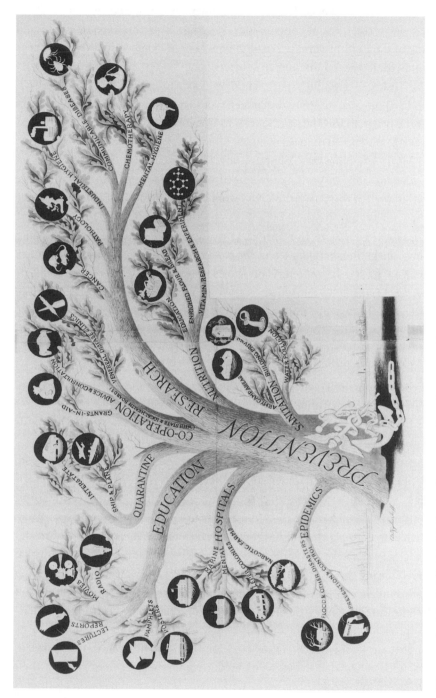

The growth of the Public Health Service became evident during World War II (1943). Department of Health and Human Services.

were reluctant to concentrate authority and power in the hands of one institution, the creation and administration of public health initiatives have often been spread over different federal agencies; these tasks have also been divided among state, local, and federal governments. American systems have often been effective in developing and implementing public health initiatives, but Public Health Service officers frequently looked to the Scandinavians, not their local or state counterparts, for guidance on how to create and implement a comprehensive sex education program. PHS officers often attributed Scandinavian success in controlling venereal disease and promoting comprehensive sex education programs to their centralized governments and social welfare systems. These successes stemmed, however, as much from these nations' homogenous population as from their centralized governments. Yet even as this obsession with the Danes, Swedes, and Norwegians led some PHS officials to advocate measures unsustainable in America, the federal government continued to develop a broadly based sex education program that enlisted not only state and local authorities but also privately funded organizations.

Public Health Service officers may have felt that their roles were constrained, at least in comparison to their European counterparts, but the surgeon general was assuming a much more powerful influence throughout this period. In 1964, Surgeon General Luther Terry released the first of what would become a series of reports on the nation's health. *The Surgeon General's Report on Smoking and Health* graphically demonstrated the dangers in smoking and ultimately resulted in labels on cigarette packs which cited a warning from the surgeon general. Both the report and the label led many Americans to become, even if only vaguely, aware of the role that the surgeon general played in creating and implementing directives for the nation's health.

Wary of the growing power of the surgeon general, Congress moved to limit the position. In the late 1960s, many of the duties associated with the surgeon general were reassigned to the secretary and assistant secretary of HEW, where they could be more directly controlled by the president. By the 1970s, the position of surgeon general had become so irrelevant that it was kept vacant while congressional leaders debated whether the position and even the Public Health Service should continue to exist as distinct entities.

All this changed when C. Everett Koop, a pediatrician with no real background in public health, was appointed surgeon general in 1981. As surgeon general during the emergence of the AIDS crisis, Koop was assured high visibility, but he also aggressively sought the spotlight to champion public health both before and independent of the AIDS crisis. More important, Koop played an active role in raising the profile of the surgeon general and the Public Health Service among his fellow Americans through such simple acts as wearing his uniform at press conferences (previous surgeons general rarely wore the uniform in public). By the late 1980s Koop was more widely recognized and trusted than any other federal appointee.[15] And when Homer Simpson, along with Principal Skinner and Abu Nahasapeemapetilon, sang "For all the latest medical poop, Call Surgeon General C. Everett Koop" on an episode of *The Simpsons* in 1993, Koop and the position of surgeon general assumed an iconic role in mainstream American culture.[16] Later surgeons general followed Koop's lead, appearing in uniform during press conferences and exploiting media such as *The Cosby Show, The Today Show,* and *Seventeen* to spread their message. Koop's own appearances as a private citizen on shows like *Da Ali G Show* further ensured that younger generations remained aware of his views. By 2007, Stephen Colbert might quip that he did not know any surgeons general except C. Everett Koop and Joycelyn Elders, but the position itself was so well known that Colbert and his colleague, Jon Stewart, could and did easily riff on the post in different shows.[17]

When Koop put on the uniform of the surgeon general in 1981, the Department of Health, Education, and Welfare and the Public Health Service were being reorganized. Following Ronald Reagan's call to downsize the federal government, the Public Health Service had closed its hospitals. With the closure of the hospitals, the mission of the Service shifted slightly as merchant marines lost their federally subsidized health care.[18] That same year, HEW became the Department of Health and Human Services (HHS), an agency devoted primarily to health. The PHS and HHS were now formally recognized as the premier arbiters for setting and enforcing standards to protect the nation's health. Neither institution could be said to be the nation's sole arbiter for shaping public health, however. The parallel growth of state and local departments of health meant that several institutions jockeyed for control of the nation's health. Local, state, and federal authorities typically worked together to combat disease and protect the nation's health, but the relationship between these varied organizations was not always a smooth one. Further upsetting this delicate balance was the fact that many public health initiatives required partnerships with schools, the military, community organizations, and a host of other institutions, all of which have had different views on public health from those advocated by the Public Health Service.

Giving Birth to Sex Education

Anthony Comstock was horrified when he walked the streets of New York City. Everywhere he looked he saw prostitutes, pornography, and advertisements for contraceptives and abortions. Comstock decided it was time to clean up the city, and in 1873 he founded the New York Society for the Suppression of Vice. But Comstock quickly realized that the vice he saw in New York could be found everywhere in nineteenth-century America. Cleaning up America would require a national, not a regional, crusade. Taking his cause to Washington, he demanded that Congress enact laws to protect Americans' purity. The same year he founded the New York Society for the Suppression of Vice, Comstock also persuaded Congress to pass an act that criminalized the selling and distribution of "obscene" materials. Recodified and reenacted several times during the twentieth century, the Comstock Act, as the law was quickly nicknamed, dramatically underscored the federal government's longstanding ability to shape Americans' behavior in their bedrooms.[19] The Act cast a long shadow and sparked fear among not only pornographers, prostitutes, and others in the sex trade but also among those who promoted sex education or the use of contraception.

Special interest groups, such as the one Comstock created in New York City, have always played a major role in shaping federal policies, and the New York Society for the Suppression of Vice was as much a product of its culture as of Comstock's forceful personality. Comstock's concerns about sexual behavior and his actions in persuading Congress to take up this cause were also far from unique. During the late nineteenth and early twentieth centuries, Americans had become increasingly agitated about sex, venereal disease, and reproduction. This agitation was central to the founding of Comstock's organization, but it also led in the opposite direction to the emergence of federally funded sex education programs.

At the turn of the century, reformers such as Comstock saw government intervention as a means of significantly improving the lives of ordinary working-class Americans. Dubbed the Progressive era, this period was characterized by both reform movements and the progressive political views of the reformers. From child labor laws to laws prohibiting the sale of alcohol or regulating industry, federal, state, and local legislators who endorsed the Progressives' agenda sponsored and enacted legislation designed to transform the American family and improve Americans' lives.

Comstock's belief that Americans' sexual morality was declining and that state and federal intervention could arrest this decline was shared by many Progressives who saw sexual immorality as a direct threat to the American family. In many ways the reformers were right to be worried about Americans' sexual morality. By the late nineteenth century both the American family and Americans' sexual behavior were in a state of flux. Before this period, working-class women overwhelmingly worked as domestic servants in situations where their employers monitored their sexual behavior. By the 1880s, growing numbers of young working-class women worked in factories, restaurants, department stores, and even offices, where they were exposed to sexual temptations unimaginable to women of their mothers' and grandmothers' generations. Within these mixed-sex workplaces, young women and men engaged in unsupervised romances. Because women were paid less than men and because they were more likely than their male counterparts to turn their wages over to their parents, many of these workers engaged in a practice known as "treating." Young men "treated" their dates to a trip to an amusement park, to a dance hall, to the theater, or to a meal. Young women reciprocated by providing sexual favors. These young women were not prostitutes, although prostitution was widespread in America at this time.[20]

Among the middle class, this period also saw a slow but gradual shift in courtship patterns. The rise of dating, which took teenagers away from the prying eyes of chaperones and lured them into dangerous places, was an especially worrisome development. Middle- and upper-class Americans still saw a woman's virginity before marriage as crucial, but young middle-class women now saw nothing very wrong in "petting," a vague term used to describe anything from kissing to more explicit forms of sexual touching.[21]

For reformers, protecting young women's virtue had never seemed so important, and a variety of organizations sprang up during this period to protect young women. These groups were all over the political spectrum. On the right, they included the Ku Klux Klan, which prioritized the protection of white women's sexuality. On the left, Progressive reformers such as those in the settlement house movement sought to protect immigrant and working-class women from sexual temptation.[22] Although women were denied the right to vote throughout much of this period, these organizations enabled women to spotlight issues ranging from unsafe working conditions to low wages. Reformers were not content with simply highlighting these problems; they also actively called upon the government to intervene on issues they saw as important to all women such as education, social welfare, morality, a living wage, pensions, and public health. Responding to pressures from these groups, the federal government, as well as its counterparts on the state level, enacted a series of maternally oriented policies during the first quarter of the twentieth century.[23]

Agitation by the General Federation of Women's Clubs was central in leading Congress to pass the Food and Drug Act in 1906. This Act brought the government directly into American homes by protecting the food Americans ate. Six years later the federal Children's Bureau was established to provide protection to children and, indirectly, families. In 1921 the passage of the Sheppard-Towner Act provided states with federal funds for maternal and child health programs as well as social welfare programs. Although the life span of the Sheppard-Towner Act was brief, the Act set a precedent for governmental measures specifically highlighting maternal and children's welfare. By the early 1920s the role of women's groups in pushing forward health legislation was so well known that physicians and legislators were openly acknowledging that "whenever they are interested in any health legislation or health education, they must [first ask] their wives . . . to bring these topics before the women's clubs . . . as that will assure their success."[24]

The Public Health Service's sex education programs originated from and reflected this impetus to protect the family through publicly funded initiatives. Although the government's first sex education campaign was directed at boys and although the creators of the materials used in this campaign were men, these programs overwhelmingly emphasized the role sex education could play in protecting women and the family.[25] Young men, boys, and soldiers were all taught that their self-control protected their future wives and children. Programs promoting sex education were, in that sense, little different from laws and programs protecting women workers and the family.

As reformers began to advocate for better sex education, public health experts echoed and endorsed the concerns that many women's groups saw in regard to declining sexual morals. There was nothing new in this warning: fears that sexual morals are declining can be found in almost any society. But in the early twentieth century several factors seemed to indicate that this was an issue of special urgency. A massive influx of immigrants, some 24 million between 1880 and 1920, led many native-born Americans to believe that their culture was under attack. Although native-born Americans' unease with different cultures led them to see immigrants as more sexually promiscuous and dangerous than native-born whites, many immigrant girls did in fact indulge in what native-born populations saw as promiscuous behavior. However, prostitution in these communities was the result of the poverty that was common in most im-

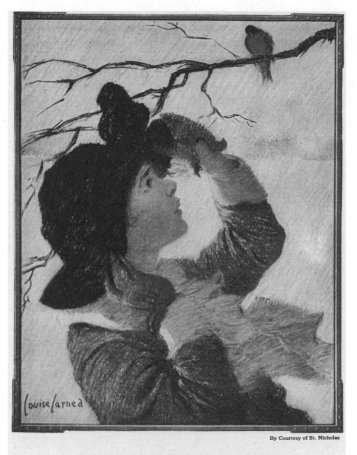

This girl may become an invalid for
life if she marries a man who has
had gonorrhea not entirely cured

Gonorrhea Causes

1. Many surgical operations upon women
2. Much invalidism among innocent wives
3. Many childless marriages

If young men and boys were sexually irresponsible, their future wives and children
would suffer. *Keeping Fit* (1918). Social Welfare History Archives, University of
Minnesota Libraries.

migrant communities, not, as many native-born Americans insisted, the immoral nature of immigrant cultures. Indignation about the supposedly high numbers of immigrant women who turned to prostitution was wildly overblown, as were rumors of "white slavers," immigrant men who lured native-born women into a life of prostitution. Progressive reformers were as susceptible to these views of immigrants as their fellow Americans, and they saw an urgent need to "Americanize" immigrants by providing them with sex education that stressed the dangers of promiscuity.

While many native-born Americans saw southern and eastern European immigrants as so foreign as to be nonwhite, the emergence of Jim Crow during the late nineteenth and early twentieth centuries also played into and reflected native-born whites' fears about the sexual behavior of nonwhites. White perceptions of African Americans, Asian Americans, and Native Americans were, and always had been, extraordinarily contradictory. On the one hand, these minority groups were routinely depicted as ugly and diseased. But on the other hand, whites also saw minority women as sexually alluring and highly promiscuous. Legislation and employment practices that reflected these fears simply exacerbated the negative stereotypes. Anti-immigration laws, intended to exclude Asian immigrants, meant that the few Asian women who arrived in the United States often came as prostitutes who were basically sold to brothel owners. Discrimination in the workplace combined with limited job opportunities meant that many African-American women who worked as domestics were more vulnerable to sexual coercion at the hands of their male employers than their white counterparts who now worked in factories, offices, and stores. Anti-miscegenation laws, which prevented interracial couples from marrying, added to these negative perceptions. Out of frustration, many of these couples simply lived together out of wedlock, a practice that fed into the widespread belief that nonwhites corrupted whites. Compounding all of these problems was the widespread poverty that existed in most minority communities. Because poverty often goes hand in hand with prostitution, divorce, and desertion, many Asian Americans, African Americans, and Native Americans engaged in sexual behavior that whites saw as immoral.

By the early twentieth century both the growing power of women's movements and the rise of a mass media pushed these fears regarding Americans' sexual behavior into the forefront of the national discussion. Newspapers, popular literature, and even films now commonly depicted men and women, immigrant and native-born, white and nonwhite, as having little concern for sexual morality. Stoked by fears that sexual promiscuity was rampant, private organizations sprang up to address the issue of sex education.

Ninety Years of Bedding Down with the Fed

Ironically, Anthony Comstock was associated with one of the earliest private organizations to promote sex education in the United States, the Young Men's Christian Association, or the YMCA, as it is more commonly known. While the Y is often viewed today as a secular organization, it began as an evangelical Protestant organization. In 1885 the YMCA organized a corps of the "White Cross Army." These were young men who were given a rudimentary form of sex education and who then took oaths of purity. Although this first form of sex education fizzled after encountering opposition from opponents within and outside the Y, it laid the groundwork for the emergence of a variety of sex education initiatives between 1890 and 1920.

In 1914 several small independent organizations combined to create a new organization dedicated to battling venereal disease. Reflecting the nation's ambivalence toward venereal disease, this organization called itself the American Social Hygiene Association (ASHA). Even as ASHA's founders pushed for openness in discussions about venereal disease, they and other Americans continued to use the euphemism "social hygiene" to refer to sexual health. Prince Morrow, a physician, became one of the first and most dynamic leaders of ASHA. Under Morrow it became the largest organization dedicated primarily to providing all Americans with good sex education. ASHA saw several issues as paramount. First and foremost, the conspiracy of silence on venereal diseases needed to be broken. Sex education should be made available in schools and through broad-reaching educational campaigns designed to change behavior. Research into the causes of sexually transmitted diseases needed to be prioritized, and the high medical costs associated with disease control needed to be contained. Finally, the nation's social, political, and religious leaders would have to speak openly about venereal disease and its impact on the nation as a whole. To accomplish these tasks, ASHA launched a massive pamphlet war. ASHA's sex education pamphlets provided some of the most detailed and most explicit sex education available in early-twentieth-century America. Some of these pamphlets were produced in-house by ASHA itself, but many were produced by the federal government and then reprinted by ASHA, which distributed them under its name.

As a private organization, ASHA lacked the funds and power to enact the agenda it advocated, and its call for a comprehensive approach to the battle against venereal disease was really directed at the federal government. By the early twentieth century, substantial precedents existed that allowed the federal government to draw upon its diverse powers to force the issue of sexually transmitted diseases into the open, to push sex education into the schools and the workplace, and to conduct research into the causes of and treatment for sexually transmitted diseases. Despite its prominence, ASHA's role in advocating this agenda was, in other words, little different from that of other smaller special interest groups. Beginning in the 1910s, the federal government aggressively took up ASHA's call and led the way in the fight against sexually transmitted diseases.

Although Americans often describe their health care system as consisting of multiple competing private institutions, the system is really a complex mosaic of private-public partnerships. These partnerships offer multiple benefits, but they also entail multiple hazards. Partnerships allow the government to develop and initiate programs on the cheap, always a benefit in a country where taxes are a hot-button political issue. Sharing resources between public and private organizations also has the benefit of distributing responsibility or, in the case of sex education, public exposure on a politically sensitive issue. But American myths about self-reliance and volunteerism as well as our emphasis on the importance of regionalism and local governance have often hampered the effectiveness of these partnerships. Even when the federal government has provided the bulk of the funding and staffing for these initiatives, organizations and communities have insisted that they, not the federal government, should control the agenda. Loud "outcries against 'federal bureaucratic meddling'" typically greet those federal officials who attempt to impose uniform standards on private organizations.[26] Complaints about "federal bureaucratic meddling" have been especially pervasive in the field of sex education.

When the federal government uses partnerships, it provides organizations with funds in the form of grants or indirect subsidies. Over the past ninety years, the organizations that have received these funds have been all over the political spectrum: conservative, progressive, secular, and religiously affiliated. At different periods, federal funds have been so prevalent that the federal government has been able to direct, or redirect, the type of sex education available to Americans.[27] Knowing that this funding may provoke an outcry, federal officials have often relied on stealth tactics when dealing with the more controversial aspects of sex education programs. These tactics have ranged from inserting provisions into bills without public debate to limiting the public's awareness of a specific program by failing to promote it widely. Whether it has been funding for religiously oriented abstinence programs in the 1990s or the promotion of condoms in the 1930s, this approach has been extremely effective in the short term. But over the past forty years Americans have come to feel that the government is funding and promoting sex education behind their backs and without their consent. This belief, more than the specific programs the federal government has sponsored, has frequently ignited Americans' anger about sex education programs.[28]

Because it has always been subject to the influence of powerful organizations and their lobbying efforts, the federal government has often found itself prey to powerful interest groups.[29] Federally funded sex education programs are no exception; these programs emerged, in the first decades of the twentieth century, from efforts by powerful women's organizations to protect women and the American family.[30] During the 1920s, as Americans became unwilling to support government initiatives to protect the family, sex education programs fell by the wayside. Ten years later, during the Great Depression, government measures designed to protect the American family came back into vogue, and sex education reemerged as a major focus of the Public Health Service. Sixty years later, when the Right agitated for a scaling back of government, sex education programs once again came under attack. Consisting of both religiously conservative voters and proponents of limited government, the Far Right agitated for the government to step aside and allow religious organizations to take over sex education programs.

Broad differences in how nongovernmental organizations and the federal government view sex education simply added to these tensions. The YMCA, the government's early partner in sex education programs, saw sex education as a matter of morality and health. Good sex education was part of the Y's broader appeal to the nation's young men to become "muscular Christians"—that is, virtuous and healthy young men. Planned Parenthood, another nongovernmental organization, saw sex education within the context of choice. Sex education should enable Americans to decide, independently, when they will have sex, how many children they will have, and when those children will be born. When promoting its own programs, the federal government has been extremely cautious about advocating a sex education agenda that may run counter to the views of a substantial segment of the American public. For this reason the government has tended to steer clear of flat endorsements of other organizations' views of sex education. In the hands of the federal government, sex education has been presented as a means of improving the nation's public health, ensuring that workers are healthy and productive, and of alleviating poverty.[31]

Although the differences between the government's views of sex education and those of private organizations may appear minor, these differences have sometimes caused open tensions between the various organizations involved in promoting sex education. More generally, however, these differences have translated into inconsistencies in how sex education programs were implemented or even what sex education should entail. Planned Parenthood's promotion of choice led that organization to promote sex education as a means of teaching Americans about reproduction and contraception, not sexually transmitted diseases. Conversely, the federal government's focus on improving Americans' health led it to prioritize not reproductive choice but the eradication of sexually transmitted diseases; in fact, a key element of the government's early sex education campaigns reflected the belief that good sexual health was tied to high fertility rates. Over time, these missions have blurred; Planned Parenthood has taken on the issue of sexually transmitted diseases, and the federal government has addressed the issue of reproductive choice. The entangled nature of privately and publicly funded sex education has, however, led to confusion about the missions and histories of federally funded sex education programs and those sponsored by private organizations.

At the local and state level, sex education programs also reflected and diverged from those developed by the federal government. On the one hand, local and state governments have heavily relied on educational materials produced by the federal government. On the other hand, communities' willingness to use these materials has differed from region to region. In America, where school districts have been and continue to be racially and economically segregated, discussions about sex education have been fractured along racial and economic lines. These divisions are often visible only when seen from a federal perspective, and yet they are central to understanding how and why sex education has become so contentious in American society. An analysis of federal efforts to promote sex education and family planning initiatives during the 1960s, for example, provides a very different insight into the conflicts. When discussing the controversies of this period, scholars have tended to look at white and predominantly middle-class communities such as Anaheim, California. There the desire to keep children "pure" led to a sharp backlash against locally sponsored sex education programs.[32] But sex education also sparked anger in very different communities. In inner cities, African-American activists saw sex education and family planning initiatives as evidence of government-sponsored genocide. Across the train tracks, working-class Catholic communities saw such initiatives as an assault on their religious beliefs.[33] When seen from the federal perspective, the history of sex education clearly reflects America's tangled history of racial and religious discrimination.

The government's strong commitment to sex education programs that serve the nation's diverse citizenry has not resulted in an unblemished record. As a white institution within a segregated society, the Public Health Service committed egregious acts such as the Tuskegee Syphilis Experiment, the infamous study of untreated syphilis in African-American men. Studies of this type often perpetuated, rather than alleviated, the problems in minority communities. They also ensured that minorities were reluctant to trust the federal government. But in a twist that demonstrates the complex nature of federal policies, the Tuskegee Syphilis Experiment developed simultaneously with innovative and broad-minded policies designed to reach all Americans, from new immigrants who spoke no English to third-generation American farmers on the Great Plains and African-American sharecroppers in the segregated South.

Seeing sex education through the lens of diversity has shaped how the government has viewed sex, reproduction, and sexually transmitted diseases. Federal officials, especially those assigned to poverty-stricken or racially segregated communities, have seen sex education as part of a broader battle against communicable diseases, poverty, racial and ethnic prejudice, and limited economic opportunities. This belief, in turn, has shaped public health officials' conviction that sex education is an issue of great urgency. But as programs and aid for the poor have come in for increasing criticism, so too has sex education come under attack.

Federal officials have never seen sex education as the sole answer to the problems of sexually transmitted diseases and unwanted pregnancies. Early on, officials insisted that sex education needed to be accompanied by laws regulating sexual behavior. Broadening sex education programs to focus on issues outside the realm of public health has meant that multiple federal agencies have become involved in the battle for sex education. Thus, the Public Health Service developed programs to educate Americans about sexuality while the Justice Department penalized those who engaged in sexual practices the government deemed dangerous. The powers of enforcement are not, of course, unique to the federal government; state and local governments have often been the primary agents in policing and criminalizing Americans' sexual behavior. However, when the federal government has chosen to enact laws of this type, their scope has been such that they impacted and shaped the behavior of millions of Americans across the country. In the 1940s, for example, the government required all young men of draft age to undergo a uniform and universal sex education program. During the same period, working with the Justice Department and the military, the Public Health Service also forced prostitutes, or those whom the government suspected to be prostitutes, to undergo mandatory sex education. Forty years later, at the height of the AIDS crisis, the government used data from tax records to bring its sex education program directly into the homes of all Americans, something private organizations could only dream about doing. Federal legislators also debated whether to impose a quarantine on AIDS patients during the early 1980s.

Eighty years before the AIDS crisis, however, the federal government was weaker than it is today, and state and local governments had a long history of passing laws related to the control of sexuality. Reflecting the widespread belief that states should take, or at least appear to take, the initiative in promoting sex education, the Public Health Service encouraged states and even private organizations such as the American Social Hygiene Association to promote federally produced sex education materials under the imprint of the state board of health or the private organization. During the Depression, power shifted away from state and local governments to the federal government, and the federal government enacted some of its most aggressive sex education initiatives in the 1930s and 1940s. The postwar expansion of the federal government under Truman and Eisenhower saw a corresponding increase in the government's actions to control venereal diseases. As the government assumed responsibility for the health care of millions of Americans under Johnson's Great Society, federal officials continued to link sex education with the battle to alleviate poverty. Arguing that unwanted children exacerbated poverty and placed undue stress upon the family, federal programs also began to educate Americans about contraception during this period. By the 1970s, the federal government's role had expanded to such a degree and its message was so broadly defined that most Americans now clearly saw the federal government as setting the tone for sex education. But the truth was that the government had always played the dominant role in sex education.

Going to War

In as early as 1917, growing numbers of Americans had come to believe that sex education was central to the nation's well-being. For those who were still ambivalent, the advent of World War I and the ensuing draft provided graphic evidence of the nation's need for sex education. High levels of venereal disease were found among recruits and "medical men working among the troops found that there [was] . . . gross ignorance and mis-education on the whole subject of sex."[34] While the creation in 1917 of the Commission on Training Camp Activities (CTCA), a program to address the recreational needs of recruits, sought to curb "the sexual impulse . . . through instruction, exercises, and wholesome entertainment," many felt that the war and its aftermath would simply exacerbate the spread of venereal disease.[35]

In the wake of the war, these concerns appeared to be validated. Throughout the 1920s the Wasserman Test, which allowed physicians to diagnose syphilis through a laboratory analysis, became increasingly common. The ability to diagnose previously overlooked or ignored cases of syphilis led many Americans to believe that syphilis was on the rise. But this was not the only problem caused by the Wasserman Test. Because the test often produced false positives, most Americans came to believe that venereal disease was more widespread than it probably was.

In a world where sexual morality was seen to be on the decline and venereal diseases seemed to be everywhere, where could Americans find good sex education and how could public health advocates ensure that people used this information properly?

CHAPTER TWO

THE PEOPLE'S WAR
1918–1926

Venereal diseases have become destructive largely because
from time immemorial a false modesty has prevented people
from discussing them frankly.
SURGEON GENERAL HUGH S. CUMMING, 1920

The youth is responsible for the generations to follow. For the
sake of his future children, he should develop self control.
KEEPING FIT, 1918

T he manager of an Illinois factory was upset. Everywhere he looked, there
was evidence of moral corruption. In his own factory, several young
women under his management had contracted venereal disease. Worse
yet, many of these women had given birth to "feeble-minded offspring." What,
the manager angrily asked, was the government doing to prevent this problem
from continuing or, even worse, escalating?

As World War I drew to a close, a growing number of letters and telegrams
asking similar questions flooded into the offices of the Public Health Service.
Over and over, the writers insisted that America's real enemy was not Germany
but rather uncontrollable young women, impulsive young men, illegitimate
pregnancies, and venereal disease. Now that the war in Europe was finally
ended, Americans demanded that the government take up what one North
Dakota farmer called the greatest work of the next generation: the promotion
of good and comprehensive sex education. Nothing more and nothing less than
a "People's War" on venereal disease and illicit sexuality was needed.[1]

Rupert Blue, the surgeon general, agreed. Over the previous forty years
changing attitudes toward sex and sexuality had brought with them the specter
of disease and illegitimate pregnancies. If aggressive action was needed to prevent both the physical and moral decay of the nation, then the Public Health
Service was more than prepared to declare war.

Congress was equally prepared to take action. In 1918, in response to an out-cry from physicians, ministers, teachers, youth leaders, and parents, it passed the Chamberlain-Kahn Act. The Act created a Venereal Disease Division with-in the Public Health Service and allowed for an immediate appropriation of $2 million to fight venereal disease, with matching funds to be provided by state legislatures. Ultimately, $4 million would be earmarked for the People's War and distributed to all but two states. Soon, public health experts told them-selves, venereal disease would be nothing more than a distant memory.

A Wave of Sex Hysteria

When Sinclair Lewis' fictional character Myra Babbit complained, "I don't understand what's come over the children of this generation . . . seems like the children today have just slipped away from all control," she spoke for an entire generation of mothers.[2] A few years before Myra's complaint, newspaper editors and Americans had insisted that a "wave of sex hysteria and sex discussion" had struck the nation.[3] As evidence, moralists never tired of pointing out that young girls now had more freedom than their mothers had had. World War I had only worsened this situation, and by 1918 a new generation was rebelling against the boundaries that had constrained their elder sisters. Upsetting as the behavior of young women was, it was young men's behavior that really alarmed the Public Health Service, politicians, teachers, youth leaders, doctors, and parents. As PHS officers and their fellow citizens grimly reminded one another, young men were inherently weak. Without the proper guidance, they were all too likely to fall prey to their worst instincts.

George was a case in point. Fundamentally, George was a good man. His friends might visit night clubs and have riotous affairs, but George was above all that. In fact, he had been sexually intimate with only three women. And those three women had been carefully chosen to ensure that they were free from dis-ease. Imagine his horror, then, when he discovered an ulcerous lesion on his genitals. Did he . . . *could* he have syphilis? Trembling with terror, George set off for the doctor. A simple exam, and the doctor confirmed his worst fears: he had syphilis.

As George lamented his fate, his doctor informed him that his situation was not as dire as he thought. "You have the good fortune to be infected with one of the diseases over which we have the most certain control," the doctor gently told him. Not only was a cure possible, its success was almost guaranteed. There was, however, one small catch. The cure, which entailed painful and repeated injections of an arsenical compound called Salvarsan, was a prolonged one with an uncertain outcome.[4] For George, who was engaged to marry a wealthy young woman, the idea of undergoing a prolonged treatment was preposterous. His doctor might refuse to sanction it, but George decided to marry—and sooner rather than later. Within a year of his marriage, George was brought face to face with his worst nightmare. His beautiful young wife became infected, and his innocent daughter was born syphilitic as well.

Although forgotten today, George's story was well known in the early twentieth century. The main character of Upton Sinclair's story *Damaged Goods*, George began life as Georges Dupont, a character in Eugene Brieux's play *Les Avaries* (The Damaged Ones). The success of Brieux's play led to its translation into English and ultimately to a retelling of the story by Sinclair in 1913. Tailor-made for the fight against venereal disease, *Damaged Goods* explored the impact of venereal disease by focusing on several stock characters: the eager young man who gives in to his sexual impulses; the good mother who wants what is best for her son but fails to teach him about sex and the benefits of virtue; the pure woman who suffers because of her husband's immorality; the innocent young child who becomes infected because of her father's promiscuity; and the hardened streetwalker who infects George out of a desire for revenge on the men who seduced and infected her.

The message of this story was clear: the wages of sin might include death for the sinner, but sexual ignorance caused even the innocent to suffer. The story did not have to unfold in this fashion, however. Passionately declaring that knowledge about sex and sexually transmitted diseases "should be spread abroad, for it is the most important knowledge in the world," George's doctor issued a plea for widespread sex education to be available "in every newspaper."[5] Only good sex education could save the Georges of the world and those whom they loved.

But what *was* good sex education?

According to the Public Health Service and its supporters in Congress and across America, good sex education rested on "accurate knowledge and a wholesome point of view." On a basic level, sex education meant teaching Americans about reproduction, the importance of caring for children, and the meaning of marriage. *Good* sex education took this a step further, by teaching that healthy sexuality was "intimately connected with the mental, physical, and moral welfare of the individual." Properly educated young adults would follow "a life of continence [or abstinence] before marriage"; after marriage, fidelity would follow naturally.[6] Fundamentally, good sex education, newspapers sternly reminded their readers, taught that "there is to be no compromise with vice in the nation-wide effort toward a higher morality."[7] This intertwining of morality and public health set the tone for both privately and federally funded sex education campaigns that emerged during the 1920s.

While the nation suffered from high rates of both venereal disease and illegitimate pregnancy, the Public Health Service's sex education program was constructed, at least in its early decades, as a war against disease, not unwanted pregnancy. The government's reluctance to discuss birth control reflected the widespread belief that children were, or should be, the welcome result of sexual intercourse, while the focus on venereal disease reflected physicians' growing confidence that they could now control infectious diseases such as syphilis and gonorrhea. Ironically, even as this new sex education campaign ignored the issue of birth control, growing numbers of Americans were endorsing and using contraceptives either to limit the size of their families or to prevent illegitimate births. But for the Public Health Service, sex education meant ensuring that Americans were healthy enough to produce healthy babies.[8]

"Men Must Live Straight If They Would Shoot Straight"

In 1917, when the United States entered World War I, concerns about venereal disease escalated. Mothers and wives wrote to President Wilson asking him to keep their boys and men "clean" and away from moral temptation. Government officials, who knew that war always sparked a rise in disease in general and venereal disease in particular, shared this concern. Just eleven days after war was declared, federal officials had established the CTCA or Commission on Training Camp Activities.

Charged with providing activities that would prevent the "moral decay" of soldiers, the CTCA developed what it called "the American Plan."[9] While European governments called for the use of medical measures to prevent the spread of venereal disease, the Americans maintained that sex education, combined with wholesome activities, could prevent an epidemic of venereal disease. By emphasizing abstinence, good sex education would provide soldiers and sailors with the necessary tools to control their sexual desire. In the words of one medical officer, "Educational measures will eventually prove effective, except in cases of utter depravity which fortunately are rare."[10]

But was depravity really rare and was the American military genuinely prepared to address this issue in its sex education programs?

An early sex education film used by the military provides some insight into the government's complex views on sexual behavior. *Fit to Fight*—after the war retitled *Fit to Win*—told the story of five soldiers and their encounters with prostitutes. Billy Hale, the film's hero, firmly refuses to have any contact with the prostitutes. Another man, a shy farm boy, exchanges a kiss with the prostitute before fleeing back to the military camp. The remaining three men, who come from varied social backgrounds, have sex with the prostitutes. Kid McCarthy, a boxer from the wrong side of the tracks, quickly returns to the camp after his encounter. There he immediately receives treatment for venereal disease. His two companions in depravity do not bother to seek medical care after they return from the brothel; they contract venereal disease, as does the innocent farm boy, who develops a cancerous lesion on his lip from the kiss of a syphilitic prostitute. Meanwhile, Billy is teased for his decision to remain chaste. Angered by this teasing, Billy proves his manliness by beating up those who mock his chastity. Deeply impressed, Kid becomes friends with Billy, and the two men vow to remain chaste.

Fit to Fight reflected several widespread beliefs. First, the film demonstrated that no one was immune to venereal disease and that prostitutes were always diseased. Second, the film sought to prove that manly men could control their sexual desires. Finally, the film argued that those who sinned by consorting with prostitutes could be redeemed—*if* they recognized the consequences of their sin and took immediate action to turn away from it.[11] Thousands of soldiers and sailors saw these films during the course of the war, and the military's willingness to provide recruits with both the knowledge and the means of preventing the spread of venereal disease indicates that military leaders were well aware that continence was more an ideal than a realistic goal.

Simply educating recruits about the dangers of venereal disease would not necessarily prevent men from turning to prostitutes. By the early twentieth century, prostitution was deeply entrenched in American life, and public health experts had long worried that prostitutes spread disease. Knowing that war always sparked a rise in sexual promiscuity, government officials quickly took aggressive action to control prostitution and, by extension, venereal disease. In the first twelve months of the war, thirty-two states passed laws that required prostitutes, or women whom government officials deemed promiscuous, to undergo compulsory testing for venereal disease. In a rare demonstration of state and federal cooperation, the U.S. Department of Justice supported and helped enforce these measures. By the end of the war, more than 18,000 women had been forcibly detained, usually in an institution that received federal funds.[12] Originally the government sought to detain and then educate these young women on the dangers of sexual promiscuity, but reformers and public health experts discovered, often to their dismay, that these young women were far from ignorant. Many of them were deliberately choosing to be sexually active.[13]

The relative brevity of America's involvement in World War I—just twenty-one months—meant that the government barely had time to develop and implement sex education programs for soldiers, sailors, and prostitutes before the war was over. Governmental officials, as well as concerned private citizens such as Prince Morrow who had long called for a nationwide sex education program, now seized the opportunity to transform these wartime programs into what would become a comprehensive and more prolonged war on sexual ignorance.

"Intelligent and Energetic Community Action"

When the boys came marching home in 1918, the Indiana State Board of Health partnered with the Public Health Service to declare "No Armistice with Venereal Diseases." Pointing out that it cost the state over $5,000 per day "to take care of the human wreckage" caused by venereal disease, state officials maintained that "men and women of sound business sense" should endorse aggressive tactics to eradicate venereal disease.[14] Indiana was not alone in advocating these measures. In nearby Iowa the state health department also urged "hard-headed business and professional men and capable women" to take action.[15] Similar cries were heard in towns and cities ranging from Middletown, New York, to Galveston, Texas.[16]

The battle against venereal disease and sexual ignorance called for a multi-faceted approach. New laws that would eradicate prostitution and other forms of illicit sexual behavior were essential in preventing the spread of venereal disease. Red light districts, which existed in every city and many towns, needed to be shut down. "Boarding houses, assignation houses, cafes, dance halls, massage parlors, amusement parks, and for-hire automobiles" were also "the refuges of clandestine prostitution," and as such these places needed to be tightly controlled. The federal government's comprehensive educational program, which educated communities on the need for these laws and the best way of garnering local support for them, provided a uniform and over-arching framework for the enactment of these laws.[17] Responding to the call, state and local officials across the nation enacted laws to control prostitution and illicit sexual activity.

The federal government's call for a nationwide educational campaign directed at young adults also struck a chord: Americans overwhelmingly believed that children and young adults needed sex education. But while parents like the fictional George Babbit sputtered that "when the proper occasion and opportunity rises" they would take their children "aside and tell [them] about— Things," many parents ruefully acknowledged that the proper occasion never seemed to arise. While parents dithered, their children were off discovering sex through what the Public Health Service called "a vast underground operation of . . . unreliable gossip . . . quack doctors and . . . lurid motion pictures."[18] Typically this "vast underground operation" reached children by the age of nine, permanently shaping their impressions of reproduction and human sexuality.

Public health experts, on both the federal and the state level, were deeply alarmed about this "vast underground operation," and they were eager to limit its influence. But differentiating pornography and sensationalism from sex education proved to be tricky, and disputes quickly developed between federal and state officials. In Iowa, for example, state officials endorsed a radically different view of sex education from that held by federal officials. The secretary of the

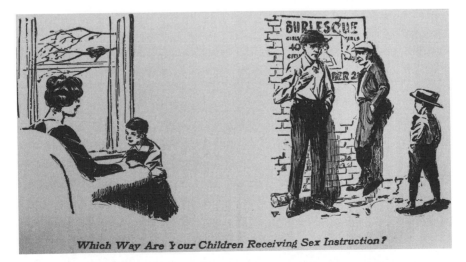

Which Way Are Your Children Receiving Sex Instruction?

In the absence of parental instruction, children learned about sex from sources the Public Health Service regarded as disreputable. *The Parents' Part* (1918). Department of Health and Human Services.

Iowa Board of Health enthused about *The Solitary Sin*, a film about a man whose obsession with masturbation leads him to kill his wife. It was, Dr. Sumner exclaimed, "the finest health film he had ever seen," and he provided opportunities for Iowans to see the film free of charge. Claude Pierce, the director of the Public Health Service's newly formed Division of Venereal Diseases, was horrified by Sumner's enthusiasm. For Pierce, *The Solitary Sin* was overwhelmingly "wrong from a medical and psychological standpoint," and it veered dangerously close to pornography. The film might cause "mental depression and a loss of confidence" among those who indulged in masturbation, Pierce argued. Films like this were the problem, not the solution to the sexual ignorance that plagued the country.[19] But to the dismay of Pierce and other PHS officers, *The Solitary Sin* was just one of many sexploitation films being shown across the nation. *The Spreading Evil, Some Wild Oats*, and similar films were just as popular and just as problematic. During the early years of the People's War, Pierce worked hard to impress upon local communities the need to vet films before they were used for sex education. By 1921, partly in response to this pressure, the federal government could point to successes. That year many Iowans reluctantly agreed that films such as *Some Wild Oats* should be pulled before they were widely circulated.[20]

Federal officials were not prepared to give up completely on the idea of sex education films, however, and a federal review board sponsored an investigation into the effectiveness of this form of sex education.[21] Films such as *Fit to Win, Open Your Eyes*, and *The End of the Road* were all characterized as good sex education, but these films could be misused. When a local movie theater advertised *Fit to Win* as a "Naked Dramatic Revelation of Sex [and] Truth Combined with a Gripping Heart Throbbing Love Story," public health experts fretted that "people go to see it in a very wrong attitude of mind."[22] Clearly, education was necessary to ensure that people viewed these films with the proper attitude.[23]

Bad sex education could be found even outside the movie theater. Medical shows and carnivals in which quacks lured people in with titillating displays and promises of quick cures presented multiple dangers: they both aroused people and misled them as to the dangers of illicit sexuality. Advertisements, books, and magazines that provided misinformation and promised quick cures were equally dangerous.

Communities needed to counter this misinformation with wholesome information about the "whole process of reproduction." "Energetic and intelligent community action" required the participation of teachers, political leaders, clergymen, youth leaders, parents, and, of course, children and adolescents. The Public Health Service called for teacher training, educational activities about the dangers of prostitution, sex education courses for working and non-working adolescents, the distribution of sex education pamphlets and placard campaigns, and, even widespread showings of the Service's first sex education films. Reflecting the views of the nation's leading progressives, sex education was now cast as a means of protecting the family through government initiatives.[24] To ensure the cooperation of communities, many of which were wary of the federal government, the Public Health Service actively encouraged state and local governments to use federal funds to reprint pamphlets and placards. Reprinted pamphlets removed any mention of the Public Health Service; in their place, state and local health departments added their own names as sponsors. To the uninitiated it appeared that the pamphlets were locally produced.

With only about seven hundred officers, the Service could not manage a public health campaign of this size on its own. Individuals needed to be recruited for this campaign, as did community organizations. By 1918, when the federal government began to promote sex education programs for all Americans, there were several precedents for this combination of private and publicly funded efforts to promote public health. The General Federation of Women's Clubs, for example, had been instrumental in assuring the passage of the Pure Food and Drug Act of 1906. In the aftermath of World War I, the General Federation of Women's Clubs, along with the Rotary Club, the American Social Hygiene Association, the Red Cross, the American Legion, the YMCA, and the YWCA, actively took up the Public Health Service's call for community action. Following the lead of state and local governments, many private organizations also reprinted federally produced pamphlets so that their organization, not the federal government, appeared as the sponsor of the material.

The media were also tapped to participate in this battle, and newspaper editors across the country published articles on the campaign and urged their readers to speak candidly about the threat posed by venereal disease. Newspapers also served as a forum for publicizing information about sex education programs.

The emergence of the government's campaign to promote sex education paralleled broader shifts in American society. During the early twentieth century, working-class and middle-class women had begun to undermine rigid Victorian moral codes by working outside the home; the independence these women gained ultimately led them to rebel against existing codes of sexual behavior.

Paralleling these shifts in women's behavior were other, equally alarming, changes. Millions of immigrants from southern and eastern Europe as well as African Americans from the South were pouring into the nation's growing cities, bringing with them a culture that white native-born Americans saw as alien and threatening. For native-born whites, Americanizing immigrants and forcing both them and African Americans to adhere to what native-born citizens saw as traditional standards of behavior became a matter of great urgency.

The greatest threat that African Americans and immigrants presented was a sexual one: as young native-born white women gained more independence, parents became increasingly fearful that immigrants and African Americans would prey upon their daughters. Protecting white women's chastity and ensuring that native-born white women married within their race or ethnic group and that they reproduced within their own race became a central goal of federally funded sex education programs. On a basic level, sex education would provide the nation's diverse citizenry with an education in sexual self-control, a trait that the nation's white Anglo-Saxon Protestant elites believed was at the heart of "their racial [and ethnic] superiority over the vulgar herd."[25] Immigrants and African Americans who aspired to move up the social ladder embraced this lesson of sexual restraint, seeing "sexual moderation and control as signs of middle-class status."[26]

While middle-class African Americans enthusiastically endorsed these efforts at sex education, segregation presented a challenge to most broadly based public health initiatives. Typically, the Public Health Service, whose commissioned corps was limited to white male physicians, ignored African-American communities when dealing with public health problems.[27] African-American leaders, however, closely linked good public health with the advancement of their race; in fact, the push to improve public health was strongly associated with the attainment of civil rights.[28] Studies developed within the African-American community argued that the legacy of slavery, as well as the continued role of racial discrimination, had led to high rates of venereal disease. In the words of one prominent African-American physician, racism and slavery had "played havoc with the home life of the colored people," and this havoc had led, in turn, to the spread of venereal disease.[29]

Whites saw the problem differently. They insisted that high rates of venereal disease among African Americans stemmed from an innate and heightened sexuality among African Americans. African-American women lured white men into temptation; African-American men preyed on white women—or so whites alleged. Antimiscegenation laws, which prohibited whites from marrying non-whites, prevented many interracial relationships, but given African Americans' supposed hypersexuality, these laws were not in and of themselves sufficient to prevent sexual encounters between the races. Protecting whites from venereal disease would require nothing less than the eradication of venereal disease among African Americans. To control what was viewed as an especially virulent epidemic of venereal diseases among African Americans and to force African Americans to endorse white notions of sexual behavior, PHS officers now crossed the color line to form partnerships with African-American institutions. The National Association of Colored Teachers, the National Medical Association, the National Association for the Advancement of Colored People, the National Urban League, and other similar organizations all worked closely with the Service to promote the federal government's sex education campaign.[30] Additionally, two leading African-American physicians, Charles V. Roman and Roscoe C. Brown, were tapped to work directly with the Public Health Service promoting sex education in African-American communities.

Stereotypes about different ethnic groups also led native-born Public Health Service officers and community officials to believe that immigrants were more sexually depraved than native-born citizens. Ugly as these stereotypes were, they held a grain of truth: immigrant communities, especially poor communities in large cities, did face daunting problems during this period. In his memoir about his childhood in New York City's tenements, *Jews without Money*, Michael Gold bitterly remembered that "Earth's trees, grass, flowers could not grow on my street; but the rose of syphilis bloomed by night and by day."[31] And when a rapist threatens Williamsburg in Betty Smith's autobiographical novel *A Tree Grows in Brooklyn*, "parents went into action. Children were told (and to hell with finding the right words) about the fiend and the horrible things he did."[32] But if tenement residents were knowledgeable about venereal disease and sexual perversions, parents in these communities tended to be as "hush-hush" about the overall nature of reproduction and human sexuality as their counterparts in wealthier communities. To address this problem, PHS officers worked with police and social workers to distribute pamphlets in these communities.[33] Translated into Yiddish, Italian, Polish, French, Greek, and a variety of other languages, these pamphlets included information on sex and venereal diseases along with more broadly defined information that the Public Health Service felt was needed to "Americanize" these new citizens.[34]

Ironically, even as native-born Americans condemned immigrants, many of whom were European, for being sexually depraved, the Public Health Service recognized that European governments were more effective at controlling venereal disease. Newspapers agreed. Pointing out that "we might well take a lesson in this from our European friends," a local paper in Delaware informed its readers that Europeans were both more honest about venereal disease and more upfront in their efforts to control it. Not everyone in xenophobic America was prepared to accept that other nations might be more effective at controlling venereal diseases, but federal officials, many of whom admired the Scandinavians' approach to public health and sex education, did encourage communities to look at and embrace Danish and Swedish attitudes toward sex education. There, communities had wholeheartedly engaged in the battle against syphilis and gonorrhea by developing both comprehensive sex education programs and establishing clinics that provided free medical care to those suffering from these diseases. In what would become almost a mantra among PHS officers over the course of the next ninety years, federal officials suggested that Americans would do well to emulate Scandinavian practices and policies.

Keeping Fit

The YMCA camp at Phantom Lake in Wisconsin had everything: nature classes, swimming, diving, boating, camping, and team sports. "I wonder if we people in Waukesha realize the value of sending our boys . . . to this wonderful camp," mused local YMCA Secretary Earl Lockman. In 1920, Waukeshans received an added value for their money when *Keeping Fit*, a new federally funded sex education program, was shown to campers. As a follow-up to the program, Frank Sherwood came out from the State Board of Health in Madison to meet with the boys and answer their questions about sex and venereal disease.[35]

Officially launched in 1918, *Keeping Fit* was the Public Health Service's opening shot in the new war on sexual ignorance. This campaign was directed at adolescent boys and young men, the group public health experts believed to be most in danger of contracting venereal disease. Produced in partnership with the YMCA, the *Keeping Fit* campaign was the brainchild of J. A. Van Dis, an immigrant with a long and distinguished career in the YMCA. Although launched from the offices of the Public Health Service, the campaign that Van Dis created and directed was really a product of the YMCA, reflecting its views on sex and sexually transmitted disease.

During the early twentieth century, the YMCA remained very much a Christian organization, but this identity was becoming less and less central to its overall mission. By the time it began working with the Public Health Service, the YMCA prided itself on its ability to reach diverse audiences. Few organizations in America had as long or as successful a track record at reaching such diverse groups.[36] Blacks and whites, rich and poor, rural and urban, native-born and immigrant, Catholics and Protestants, and even Christians and non-Christians were all targeted with the Y's new message emphasizing the link between personal morality and health.

If any organization could make sex education acceptable to the more conservative elements of American society, it was the YMCA. That said, the Public Health Service and the Y both knew that even the most conservative sex education program could cause offense. However, federal officials rather naively believed that they could limit opposition to their sex education programs by pitching their initial campaigns at adolescents and adults, as opposed to young children. This decision stemmed from the belief that placating conservatives was crucial to the success of *Keeping Fit* and the entire People's War. Unfortunately, it proved to be the first in what would be a series of missteps by the Service.

Long before it launched the People's War, the Public Health Service had been aware that most Americans wanted sex education aimed at young children, and PHS officials believed that sex education should begin when a child was four or five.[37] But even as the PHS acknowledged this, it was driven by fears that conservatives would attack any form of federally sponsored sex education. To prevent or at least limit potential criticism, the PHS aimed low. *Keeping Fit*, its first sex education campaign, was targeted at boys between the ages of fourteen and twenty-one, boys who already knew the facts of life.

Because most American boys in 1918 left school at fourteen or fifteen, reaching adolescents, most of whom were dispersed across the American workforce, required creativity and effort. Eager to do their share, Rotary Clubs partnered with the federal government and YMCA officials to ensure that businessmen and employers promoted the program. Foremen were encouraged to become familiar with the program as well. Bragging that they had shown *Keeping Fit* in the "dingy basements of factories and . . . in luxuriously furnished directors' offices of banks," the Public Health Service also displayed the exhibit in city halls, churches, workplaces, and community centers.[38] Attendance at these programs was voluntary, but *Keeping Fit* reached several million working boys in its first few years.

Reaching boys still in school also presented difficulties. The highly decentralized nature of the American school system prevented the federal government from issuing a flat mandate requiring all American schools to mount a sex education program. Instead, the Public Health Service offered financial incentives as well as access to materials to schools that were interested in promoting *Keeping Fit*. Surprisingly, this technique actually turned out to be fairly successful as thousands of school districts opted to use *Keeping Fit*, clear evidence of a very real demand for good sex education. Teachers were especially enthusiastic. As one exclaimed, "I am glad that the Government has taken [sex education] up." Parents were also pleased with the program. After his son viewed *Keeping Fit* in his school, one father told the PHS that the program "was worth $500 to my boy."[39]

Responses to *Keeping Fit* varied widely and often reflected regional stereotypes. In a sharp contrast to today, the South was most enthusiastic about sex education. This enthusiasm stemmed from the widespread belief that venereal disease was more prevalent among African Americans than whites. Southerners did not, of course, have a monopoly on racist beliefs or on the implementation of racist policies; however, given the South's large African-American population, officials there were more apt to create policies reflecting such prejudices. In the case of sex education, racist beliefs, combined with the desire to protect both the African-American labor force as well as those whites who engaged in sexual encounters with African Americans, resulted in an extremely progressive attitude toward sex education. But in Boston and other northeastern cities, local authorities saw the issue quite differently. Fearing that the use of public funds to provide sex education would offend the Northeast's large Catholic population, city officials in Boston and elsewhere often resisted showing *Keeping Fit* and similar programs.[40] Despite this resistance, *Keeping Fit* reached several million schoolboys during 1918 and 1919, with a promise of wider dissemination in the coming years.

But what exactly were those who saw *Keeping Fit* viewing? Did *Keeping Fit* alter American boys' understanding of sexuality and sexually transmitted diseases?

Keeping Fit consisted of fifty slides or posters. Each poster contained an image accompanied by a brief text. The exhibit could be shown using lantern slides, posters, or even an illustrated pamphlet that boys could read in the privacy of their own homes. Ideally, boys viewed the exhibit in a public setting where a male lecturer, provided by the YMCA and paid for by the Public Health Service, was available to answer questions. In remote rural areas, limited funding, combined with the difficulty of collecting large numbers of boys in one place, meant that public exhibits with lecturers were rare or nonexistent. Boys in these communities were expected to read the pamphlet at home. And read it at home they did. After reading the pamphlet, boys from rural states and territories such as Nevada and Alaska often wrote in to the Public Health Service asking for additional information and advice.

Keeping Fit exploited American boys' love of athletics by linking sexual health with physical fitness. The exhibit also highlighted manly men such as train conductors, soldiers, and presidents. As an athlete, former soldier, and president, Theodore Roosevelt delivered a trifecta, and the story of his transformation from an asthmatic weakling into a rough-riding cowboy served to remind boys that sexual, and physical, health required effort and self-control. Implicit in this imagery was the assumption that physical and moral strength were linked, and that only physical and moral weaklings gave in to sexual temptation.

The idea of self-control, control of the body and mind, was central to the *Keeping Fit* program. The terms *self-control* and *will-power* were constantly repeated in the text. Boys were urged to "take no liberties." Over and over the text drove home the point that a lack of control leads to disease, decay, and, ultimately, death. This message was already familiar to many Americans, as it had been a central component of the antialcohol, antinarcotic, and antituberculosis movements. By emphasizing the idea of control, the creators of *Keeping Fit* balanced the more shocking aspects of their program (an open discussion of venereal disease) with a more conservative message (a call to reprioritize marriage). Obviously this emphasis on sexual control did not totally eradicate the shock presented by the Public Health Service's candid discussion of venereal disease, but it did enable federal officials to discuss venereal disease in a manner that would gain the support of the more conservative elements of American society.

For the modern viewer of *Keeping Fit*, the most striking aspect of the program is its almost complete failure to discuss reproduction or sexually transmitted diseases. In part this reticence to speak candidly stemmed from the belief that explicit discussions of sex were vulgar and characteristic of sexually degenerate cultures. In other words, simply by avoiding detail and frankness, *Keeping Fit* endorsed and reflected the middle-class views of sexuality that its creators believed were central to preventing the spread of venereal disease.[41]

If *Keeping Fit* avoided explicit discussions of sexuality, the program did include substantial information on the proper way to eat a meal, the value of cleanliness, and the importance of drinking plenty of water. Less substantial was the exhibit's discussion of the importance of reproduction and the need to avoid sexually trans-

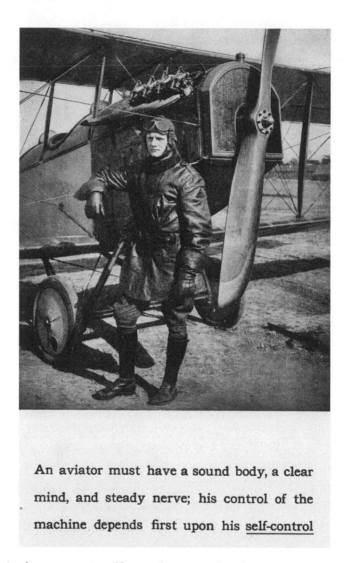

An aviator must have a sound body, a clear mind, and steady nerve; his control of the machine depends first upon his self-control

Encouraging boys to exercise self-control was central to the *Keeping Fit* program. *Keeping Fit* (1918). Social Welfare History Archives, University of Minnesota Libraries.

mitted diseases through self-control. It was almost as though the Service recognized that the boys viewing the exhibit already knew the facts of life. And the truth was, of course, that many of these boys *did* know these "facts." If nothing else, the comments that boys submitted to lecturers after viewing the exhibit— which ranged from earnest questions as to whether masturbation really damaged one's health to suggestions that their *younger* brothers would better benefit from the exhibit—all indicated that the exhibit did not answer adolescents' questions.[42] This failure to reach and educate boys most in need of good sex education was a troubling one. Federal officials genuinely wanted to provide Americans with accurate and "scientific" information about sexuality without offending anyone, but when they attempted to translate this belief into practice, they discovered that it was a difficult if not impossible task. Fundamentally, the promotion of scientific information clashed with the promotion of "moral values."

This tension between science and morality could be found throughout *Keeping Fit*, but it was most evident in discussions about masturbation. During the nineteenth century, clergymen, parents, and physicians had insisted that masturbation caused blindness, insanity, and even infertility. By the early twentieth century, scientific practitioners overwhelmingly rejected these views of masturbation as wrong. In scientific terms this was all well and good, but within the moral climate of 1918, this issue presented a serious bind for the Public Health Service. If masturbation did not pose a risk to health, what was to prevent boys from engaging in this morally unacceptable behavior?

Masturbation, the Public Health Service admitted, might not itself cause blindness, insanity, or infertility. But boys who engaged in this type of behavior lacked self-control and were likely to find themselves unable to resist temptation later on. And, as everyone knew, boys who were unable to resist temptation became men who visited prostitutes and engaged in sexual relationships with immoral women. These men ultimately contracted venereal disease, and it was venereal disease that caused blindness, insanity, and infertility. It was convoluted reasoning at best, but the Public Health Service believed it to be highly effective nonetheless. Given the fact that in 1996, some seventy years after the PHS first skirted this issue, a surgeon general who failed to condemn masturbation found herself embroiled in a media frenzy over the issue, the Public Health Service's decision to punt on this issue in 1918 was understandable. Early-twentieth-century Americans almost universally viewed masturbation— in fact, *any* form of nonreproductive sex—as morally wrong. This did not mean, of course, that they did not engage in this type of behavior. They did. However, no one wanted the federal government to advocate "immoral" behavior, and in the eyes of most Americans, anything short of condemnation of masturbation amounted to tacit approval.

Emphasizing morality over science led the Public Health Service into even more costly mistakes. Hoping to prevent all sexual encounters outside of marriage, the PHS did little to provide Americans with detailed information about the prevention and treatment of venereal disease. For example, although the PHS and most physicians were aware that condoms prevented venereal disease, the PHS did not provide Americans with this information. Instead, it emphasized continence or abstinence as the only effective form of prevention. Additionally, although aware that arsenical compounds could, when taken over a prolonged period, cure venereal disease, the PHS did not make this information widely available, even as its own hospitals and clinics treated those suffering from venereal disease in this fashion. This decision not to advertise or even highlight a cure for venereal disease may have stemmed from the Service's belief that open discussions of cures or preventive measures would cause people to throw caution to the wind.

As part of its attempt to promote sex education as a community effort, the Public Health Service encouraged lecturers and organizations to alter the program to respond to different needs. For its creator, Van Dis, this meant that lecturers could "take the Government material and ... Christianize the message."[43] Van Dis was savvy enough not to make this statement publicly or even in private to the PHS officers with whom he worked. Yet this was a sentiment that most PHS officers, the majority of whom were Christian, might well have happily endorsed. In fact, for most early-twentieth-century Americans, even the most enlightened, the program's linking of Christian morality and sexual health would have been viewed as a positive element of the campaign. But while acceptable and even popular in 1918, this overt inclusion of Christian images would come to dog later sex education campaigns, as the nation became both more diverse and less Christian.

While the Public Health Service had always intended communities to alter sex education materials to fit their needs, its officers were a bit displeased when they discovered just *how much* communities changed the program. When several schools in California decided to omit exhibit panels that dealt with venereal disease, the PHS angrily threatened to cut off funds for these schools. Halfway across the country, schools such as Centralia Township High School in Illinois simply omitted panels they disliked and casually notified the PHS after they had received the necessary funding to support the presentation of the materials. Similarly, private organizations altered *Keeping Fit* to reflect their own views on sex education. The nation's most prominent sex education organization, the American Social Hygiene Association, reprinted *Keeping Fit*, adding more panels to the original twenty-eight and releasing this revised version with its own name and logo. In general the PHS took a pragmatic approach to these alterations. In 1918, PHS officers saw themselves as laying the groundwork for an ongoing war on sexual illiteracy, and they were prepared to pick their battles. If allowing communities to alter its carefully crafted program was what it took to promote sex education, then the PHS was willing to accept alterations that did not substantially negate or dilute its message.

Allowing communities to modify programs to reflect local values was in many ways the only approach the Public Health Service could take, given the nation's growing diversity. Ultimately this tactic would lead the PHS to begin tailoring different and unique messages for specific groups. African Americans, for example, would receive materials highlighting images of African Americans. Immigrants would not only receive materials in their own language, they would also receive materials that reflected the values of their culture. Women would receive different messages from men. This eagerness to adopt an array of approaches foreshadowed what would ultimately be regarded as a fundamental component of good public health education: a willingness to craft unique messages that reflected the cultures and needs of specific groups.

On the surface this flexibility was an incredible leap forward for public health. However, this flexibility also had a downside. Because communities altered programs such as *Keeping Fit*, the Public Health Service was never able to issue a uniform sex education program directed at *all* Americans. Throughout the twentieth century, government-sponsored sex education campaigns would consist of multiple messages using multiple media. As a result, these campaigns tended to be extremely expensive—always a liability for a government-funded program. More disturbing still, because communities routinely modified the government's materials, the PHS found it impossible to determine which methods were truly successful and why. Unable to pinpoint the most successful aspects of its programs, the PHS often found it difficult to prove to Congress and the American taxpayer that the programs worked and, more important, that they deserved increased funding.[44] In the long term this approach would also suffer as Americans are often reluctant to support programs they do not see as benefiting them directly. As sex education programs were increasingly tailored to address specific audiences, and as the threat of venereal disease began to lessen for many Americans, taxpayers began to question the need to support sex education programs.

Expanding the People's War

One night in rural Maine a woman lecturer made a long and lonely trek to the local schoolhouse. By the time she reached the school, it was filled to overflowing. For an hour, lit only by a "kerosene lamp on the teacher's desk and the occasional flare of a man's pipe," the woman lectured the community on "how venereal diseases menace even the rural family." Halfway across the country in Ada, Oklahoma, the local paper noted with pride that the "work of stamping out . . . social diseases in Oklahoma is going on with unabashed vigor on the part of the U.S. Public Health Service."[45] All over America, communities had embraced the People's War.

Reflecting its belief that the "crusade against ignorance" would require a "wide use of pamphlets, lectures, motion pictures and exhibits,"[46] the Public Health Service created a program that was as diverse as the nation. Between 1918 and 1920 the PHS flooded the nation's farming communities, towns, and cities with "pamphlets, lectures, motion pictures, and exhibits." During the first two years of the crusade, over 1.4 million people flocked to see a sex education film endorsed by the PHS. During that same period, over 5,000 businesses established some sort of venereal disease program, and a health-mobile, equipped with two PHS officers and a variety of sex education films, traveled across the nation. Thirty-one national conferences of educators were held, and best of all, over 22 million pamphlets were distributed, to groups ranging from the Modern Woodsmen of America, a fraternal benefits company, to the National Association of Teachers in Colored Schools.[47]

Ministers also took up the cause. February 2, 1919, a Sunday, was declared Social Hygiene Day, and ministers preached sermons stressing the role of continence and fidelity as a means of preventing venereal disease. From Arkansas to New York, club women gathered to make a "careful study of the subject" and to work to "interest [others] in Social Hygiene."[48] But most important, schoolteachers and principals began to work closely with the Public Health Service to promote sex education.

During the early 1920s, as the number of adolescents remaining in school increased,[49] Public Health Service officers upped the ante. They developed *The Science of Life*, a sex education program intended specially for adolescent girls. They also reformatted *Keeping Fit*, replacing images of white boys with African-American boys so that the program could be used in African-American communities. And they stepped into the twentieth century by producing two films for

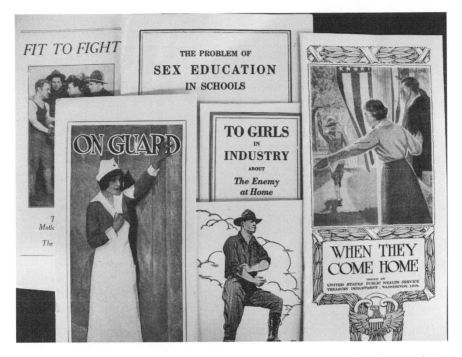

Pamphlets were specifically directed at different constituencies. Author photograph/
Department of Health and Human Services.

use in the classroom. Films, the PHS felt, had the potential to be an effective educational medium; however, they could cause undue excitement, always a negative for a serious sex education program. To downplay this excitement, the PHS rejected the use of a storyline and chose chillingly scientific titles—*Personal Hygiene for Boys* and *Personal Hygiene for Girls*—for its films. Released in 1924, these films consisted of animated but silent versions of the illustrations in *Keeping Fit* and *The Science of Life* accompanied by subtitles.

While in many ways a ground-breaking effort, the films were mind-numbingly dull. Worse yet, they were also the victims of poor timing. In 1927 the release of *The Jazz Singer*, the first movie with sound, instantly made all silent films obsolete and dated. Of course, as all Americans know, the use of out-dated images has never prevented a school district from using readily available films or textbooks. But widespread as this practice may be, it has never been an especially successful approach to education. Teenagers tend to be so aware of subtle changes in popular culture and fashion that reaching them almost always requires the use of images and words that reflect current fashion. Judged by this standard, both *Personal Hygiene for Boys* and *Personal Hygiene for Girls* were disasters. In fact, by the time these films began to be shown widely in the late 1920s and 1930s, teenagers across America must have viewed the silent images of sedate girls in long dresses and athletic boys in knickerbockers as laughably irrelevant.

The Fog of War

Seeking "to make people good by science,"[50] the People's War sought to validate traditional moral codes by giving them a veneer of science. Despite their insistence that they were rejecting the "false modesty" of previous generations,[51] Public Health Service officers actively endorsed traditional images and views of sexuality—just as these images and views were declining in American society. Small wonder, then, that many Americans, living lives very different from the model endorsed by the PHS, found it hard to become enthusiastic about the campaign during its later years.

The Public Health Service's reliance on volunteer organizations also doomed the campaign. With *Keeping Fit*, the PHS had established a partnership with the highly professional YMCA. While the YMCA used volunteers, their work for the PHS was done by salaried workers whose expenses were reimbursed. The deep coffers of the YMCA allowed the organization to match and sometimes exceed the funds provided by the PHS, which meant that the Y could stage repeated showings of *Keeping Fit* and advertise them widely. Unfortunately, the Public Health Service's reliance on other volunteer organizations was much more problematic. Organizations such as the General Federation of Women's Clubs (GFWC), for example, could not provide any financial support for these programs—and financial support was crucial, as mounting PHS-sponsored programs often entailed renting halls and lantern projectors and paying the travel expenses of lecturers. Additionally, because the GFWC and similar organizations were staffed by volunteers, many of whom held full-time jobs, they were unable to provide staff who could devote their time to this issue.

Following the passage of the Chamberlain-Kahn Act, Americans and their congressmen had been eager to provide financial support for sex education. But Americans have always had a notoriously short attention span. During the late 1920s, as interest in venereal disease waned and new concerns came to the fore, funding for these programs dramatically declined. Starved of funds, the Public

Health Service ceased both to produce new pamphlets and to provide funding to communities interested in tackling venereal disease. PHS materials did not, however, disappear. Relegated to the dusty cupboards of classrooms and community centers, these materials continued to be used, although only sporadically, throughout the late 1920s and early 1930s.

The sidelining of the government-sponsored People's War should not be interpreted as evidence of the ineffectiveness or unimportance of this campaign. The program laid the groundwork for several important innovations in both the structure of government-sponsored public health campaigns and approaches to sex education. In creating this campaign, the Public Health Service firmly placed sex education in the hands of the government. More important, though, the PHS set a new standard for the way in which public health campaigns could be run: by envisioning health education as an ongoing and continuous effort, PHS officers and their partners challenged contemporary views of health education as a stopgap measure intended to address specific or regionally focused health crises. While it is true that the campaign did not become a permanent part of the American landscape in the way in which its creators had hoped, the program was the first and crucial step in what can now be seen as a continuous campaign by the American government to educate the public on sexuality and sexually transmitted diseases.

CHAPTER THREE

BATTLING THE MAD DOG
1927–1940

There has been a persistent feeling that blundering humans should not discuss sex lest they corrupt and spoil it.

SURGEON GENERAL THOMAS PARRAN, 1940

The use of the rubber (condom) during sexual intercourse . . . protects both the man and the woman.

SYPHILIS: ITS CAUSES, ITS SPREAD, AND ITS CURE, 1937

W hen Dizzy Malone burst into his office, the District Attorney couldn't help himself. " 'Dizzy Malone,' he gasped, 'the same, gorgeous body and all!' " A "jane with a . . . red past," Dizzy "went to men's heads." She was every adolescent boy's dream of a bad girl. Yet despite her appeal, this blonde bombshell had her limitations; she was, after all, nothing more than the creation of a pulp fiction writer.[1]

As a fictional character, Dizzy lived a wild life in which guns, illegal drinking, and crime played prominent roles. To most American women this lifestyle was completely alien, though to some it had familiar elements. Dizzy's roadster, her forays into wild jazz clubs, and her free and easy relationships with men all marked her as a flapper, one of the new women who had emerged during the 1920s. Throughout the 1920s and into the 1930s, these young women rebelled against Victorian conventions, rejecting their chaperones and moving, in the words of one historian, from the front porch swing to the back seat of a car.[2]

The sexual revolution that these young men and women initiated spread rapidly. By the late 1920s even such quintessentially heartland towns as Muncie, Indiana, had felt the seismic shift of this revolution. There, indignant mothers complained about their teenagers' behavior. "Six girls organized a party and invited six boys and they never got home until three in the morning," one distraught Muncie mother exclaimed in shock.[3] Teenagers' views on the situation differed. As Maudie Mason, the heroine in a series of books who later went on to fame as a character on a radio show, put it, "You would think parents would get over this idea that the age of consent means theirs." For Maudie and her real-life counterparts, the "men who want a girl to be a regular Sweet Adelaide" were "prehistoric."[4]

If teenagers scorned Sweet Adelaides, what did they really want?

With over half of Muncie's teenagers admitting that they engaged in "petting parties," parties that featured kissing and light sexual touching, the answer was obvious. For public health experts, the answer was also deeply alarming. As the sexual revolution snaked its way across the country, they knew that Americans remained appallingly ignorant about sex and sexually transmitted diseases.

The People's War, begun with such fanfare and such high hopes in 1918, had staggered into oblivion. In its wake had come the Depression, poverty, and rising rates of venereal disease. Within five years of the program's launch, states had begun to cut back on their sex education programs. By the mid- to late 1920s, the educational directors of state health departments, who had survived the first round of budget cuts, became jobless as a second or even third round of cuts occurred. The ten-year anniversary of the People's War found states struggling to continue their sex education programs as federal funds evaporated. Lacking a structured and well-financed educational program to provide an impetus, requests for sex education materials slowed to a trickle. Worse yet, the movies produced by the Public Health Service at the height of the People's War were now so dated and worn that they were no longer usable. For commissioned officers of the PHS and for state and local authorities, the situation looked bleak indeed.[5] But all this began to change in 1932 when Franklin D. Roosevelt was elected to the presidency.

In the half-century before the New Deal, state, not federal, legislators had been at the forefront of banning or regulating personal behavior, such as the consumption of alcohol or the operation of brothels. In fact, before 1933, state and local governments expended greater sums on public welfare and assumed more responsibilities in this regard than the federal government.[6] Reflecting this view, state and local governments saw themselves as being on the front lines of the venereal disease crisis; it was their laws and their policing that would control this crisis. Throughout the 1910s and 1920s, the federal government had agreed. Pamphlets and brochures produced by the federal government often spoke of the need for *communities* to become actively engaged in the battle against venereal disease and to pass laws regulating sexual behavior. In the Northeast, for example, fears of offending Boston's sizable Catholic population had led the federal government to pull its punches during the People's War. With the full knowledge of federal officials, local officials in Boston and other northeastern cities had appeased Catholic conservatives by watering down the *Keeping Fit* program. The federal government's reluctance to set the public health agenda during this period is somewhat surprising. The late nineteenth century had been characterized by a series of cases and precedents, all of which indicated that the Public Health Service could overrule state and local officials in the event of a public health crisis. Yet the newness of these precedents, combined with very real concerns that state and local officials would resent federal interference, continued to shape federal policies in the two decades before the New Deal.

The primacy of state laws and initiatives was also demonstrated by the activities of nongovernmental public health experts. Throughout the 1920s and well into the 1930s, public health advocates from organizations such as the American Social Hygiene Association needed to take their initiatives to forty-eight state legislatures, a time-consuming and frustrating process. Under Roosevelt, the federal government expanded and became more directly engaged in the battle against venereal disease, explicitly telling states to follow its initiatives and policies. The federal government also took direct control over financing of sex education; previously, all states had received equal allocation of funds, but now federal officials assessed a state's needs before allocating funding. This ultimately led to a more uniform approach to controlling venereal disease, but it also meant that sex education programs could run afoul of claims that the federal government was "meddling" in local affairs.

Prescribing Parran

As governor of New York, Roosevelt had appointed a career Public Health Service officer, Thomas Parran, to be commissioner of health for the state of New York. Parran, a Marylander and a Catholic, was a passionate advocate for a range of public health issues, but he reserved his greatest efforts for the battle against venereal disease. During the 1920s Parran was the director of the Venereal Disease Division of the Public Health Service. In this capacity Parran developed an in-depth understanding of the impact these diseases had on different communities and the problems that emerged when funding for sex education was slowly strangled. Moving from the PHS to become the commissioner of health for New York State in 1930 provided Parran with a perfect opportunity to expand on this knowledge. New York State, which was home to the nation's largest city as well as a range of midsized cities and rural communities, graphically illustrated the extent to which sexually transmitted diseases found their way into both rural and urban areas.[7] When President Roosevelt tapped Parran to become his surgeon general in 1936, he did so knowing that almost no other public health expert knew, or cared, as much about venereal disease as Parran did. In accepting the nomination, Parran believed that he could finally force the entire nation to prioritize the battle to contain venereal disease.

Parran had spent the formative years of his public health career fighting venereal disease, and he began his tenure as surgeon general with clear-cut and very strong beliefs about venereal disease, which he termed "the mad dog of communicable diseases."[8] In many ways Parran's views and past experiences meant that he tended to initiate and use approaches similar to those of his predecessors. But Parran's particular passion for the battle against venereal disease also led him to publicize the issue more aggressively than any other previous surgeon general. In response, Congress expanded funding for programs the Public Health Service sponsored—a crucial step forward for federally funded sex education programs.

Several other changes during Parran's tenure also radically transformed the battle against venereal disease. In the mid-1940s the creation of the Communicable Disease Center, as it was then called, centralized the tracking of diseases. As the CDC began determining rates of venereal disease, the Public Health Service was forced to become more accountable for the success or failure of its educational programs.[9] Although many privately funded organizations later created independent programs to monitor and assess rates of infection, the federal government was the first to tie its sex education programs directly to large-scale epidemiological studies of venereal disease.

Even before the CDC began assessing rates of venereal disease, the introduction of sulfa drugs in the 1930s and then of penicillin in the mid-1940s had dramatically altered treatment for and attitudes toward sexually transmitted diseases. But while penicillin was widely touted as a miracle drug, it had its limits. It did nothing to assist in the emerging war against "sexual promiscuity" and its corollary: illegitimate pregnancy.

Low Moral Standards

Felix Underwood, the executive director of the State Board of Health in Mississippi, told a chilling story in 1938. One of his former patients had first shot his wife and then his mother-in-law. Reeling from what he had done, the man then turned the gun on himself. When the gun failed to fire, he committed suicide by jumping out a window. What had caused the tragedy? "Well," Underwood explained, "the papers had a good deal to say about domestic trouble and jealousy. [But] I knew that the man had developed a homicidal mania from syphilis." The issues precipitating the event were complex, but one fact was clear: an increase in federal funding for sex education, along with cheaper treatments, would prevent this type of tragedy in the future.[10]

No one knew the importance of federal involvement better than Underwood. Mississippi, Underwood's home state, ranked at the bottom of almost every gauge of public health. Pellagra, tuberculosis, malaria, hookworm, and a variety of other diseases plagued the state's residents. Compounding the problem were high maternal and infant mortality rates and poor doctor-patient ratios. Most worrisome of all were the rapidly rising rates of venereal disease. Developing and implementing good public health initiatives would require money, but the state's longstanding policies of racial and class segregation meant that few voters and even fewer state officials were prepared to allocate funding for programs that benefited the state's poorer residents, many of whom were African American. Throughout the late 1920s and 1930s, Underwood courted the state's wealthier residents, cajoling them into understanding that improvements in public health would benefit all Mississippians. Ultimately some of the state's more prominent and more progressive business owners came to acknowledge the role good public health programs played in creating a healthy workforce, but it was an uphill battle.[11] If Underwood and his colleagues in states with similar policies of discrimination and disenfranchisement were ever to make progress in the war against venereal disease, federal funds and federal support would be needed.

Three years before Underwood told his story at a packed Senate hearing, the enactment of the Social Security Act in 1935 had made his plea somewhat less urgent. The Act had provided some funding for public health, with $8 million being released in 1936.[12] Given the dire state of public health funds before 1935, the Act provided little more than the basics needed to reinvigorate the People's War. Surgeon General Parran wanted more. In 1938 he spearheaded a movement demanding that Congress increase funding to fight venereal disease and sexual ignorance. A series of testimonies such as Underwood's ensured passage of the Act. Following its enactment, the National Venereal Disease Control Act poured $15 million into the Public Health Service's campaign against sexual ignorance. Funding escalated over a three-year period, with $3 million being made available the first year, $5 million the second, and $7 million the third. Learning from its mistakes, the Public Health Service pushed for greater control over the allocated money. After 1938, rather than provide equal funds to all communities and states, the PHS was finally able to divert money to those communities most in need of financial assistance.[13]

Finding funds for this new public health campaign was a necessary first step. However, other problems faced public health experts and community activists as they worked to reinitiate the war on venereal disease. American attitudes regarding venereal disease needed to be radically transformed if the war was to be fought effectively. Fundamentally, Americans needed to become comfortable with discussing syphilis and gonorrhea more openly.[14]

Both before and after he became surgeon general, Parran aggressively broke what he and other public health experts insisted was a national taboo on the very use of terms such as *syphilis*, *gonorrhea*, and *venereal disease*. To push Americans into becoming more aware of these diseases, Parran published articles about venereal disease in some of the nation's most popular magazines. The most famous of these was a 1937 article in the normally staid *Ladies Home Journal*. In the article Parran encouraged Americans to confront the venereal disease crisis with an assessment of the "dastardly" way this "microbe gangster sneaks back out of his hiding." For those who may have missed his point, Nancy Hale's accompanying story "The Blue-Muslin Sepulchre" provided a gruesome reminder of the dangers of ignorance. Reflecting the same themes that had been highlighted in *Damaged Goods*, Hale's story focused on a doctor's failure to notify a family of the father's syphilis and the consequences of this failure for the health of all members of the family, particularly the two daughters.[15] The editors of *Reader's Digest* also jumped on the bandwagon by allowing Parran to speak directly to their readers. In 1937 Parran even published a book. Aided by Parran's high-profile status as the surgeon general, *Shadow on the Land*, which spoke frankly about syphilis, became a surprise bestseller.

On the rare occasions when Parran encountered opposition, he turned the opposition to dramatic effect. After Columbia Broadcasting refused to allow then–New York State Commissioner of Health Parran to use the word *syphilis* on radio, Parran refused to appear on the show, dramatically resigned from his position on the National Advisory Council on Radio in Education, and initiated a "vigorous cry against radio censorship." These actions provoked as much attention as a simple discussion of venereal disease would have garnered, if not more.[16] Yet Columbia's refusal to allow him to speak publicly about syphilis should not have come as a surprise to Parran; two years before Columbia's refusal, the National Broadcasting Company had denied the same opportunity to Parran's colleague, John Rice, the New York City commissioner of health. Both organizations later confessed that they feared that "a family or mixed group might be shocked by mention of syphilis" and "denounce" them.[17]

In 1934, as New York State Commissioner of Health Parran began demanding the right to discuss venereal disease openly, the film industry was agreeing to submit to a form of censorship. That year the Hays Code, which regulated the film industry, was implemented. Developed in 1930 by a Catholic priest, the Hays Code was simply a set of guidelines for film producers. At heart, the code was intended to ensure that no film would be produced that would "lower the moral standards of those who see it." Sex scenes were rigidly censored, and the code explicitly stated that "sex hygiene and venereal diseases are not subjects for motion pictures." Officially, the code lacked any method of enforcement. However, producers' fears of a boycott by Catholic, and even Protestant, theatergoers in Boston, Chicago, and other cities led filmmakers to rework their films to reflect these guidelines.

The code was a mixed blessing for the Public Health Service. During the 1910s and 1920s, Hollywood had churned out sexploitation films under the guise of sex education. *The Solitary Sin*, for example, had claimed to educate viewers on the dangers of masturbation through its story of a man who becomes so addicted to masturbation that he kills his wife. While the PHS was not prepared to say that masturbation was healthy or normal, its officers were concerned that films such as these led to possibly harmful feelings of guilt and shame. Much to the relief of the PHS, the Hays Code basically banned the production of films of this type as well as less blatantly sexual films such as those written and produced by Mae West. However, the Hays Code also made it more difficult to produce, and to promote as good sex education, films that treated syphilis and gonorrhea in a serious fashion. In 1934 the film version of Somerset Maugham's book *Of Human Bondage* became an early victim of the Code. Although based on a book that had candidly discussed syphilis, the film was forced to skirt the issue completely by having its main character develop tuberculosis rather than syphilis. In 1940, when Warner Brothers worked with the PHS to produce *Dr. Ehrlich's Magic Bullet,* a film about Paul Ehrlich's discovery of an effective treatment for syphilis, reviews of the film noted that the filmmakers, "with a word of warning from the Hays office," created a film in which the disease is rarely mentioned by name.[18]

This push toward censorship did not accurately reflect Americans' complex views on sex and venereal disease. Throughout the 1930s public response to Parran's candid and aggressive discussions of syphilis was overwhelmingly positive. The *Ladies Home Journal,* for example, had received hundreds of letters in response to Parran's article, only one of them negative. Boasting that "discussion of the article [is] . . . everywhere," *Reader's Digest* found itself in the enviable position of making money when organizations and individuals demanded over a quarter of a million reprints of Parran's article.[19] When a 1938 Gallup poll asked if they would favor the distribution of information about venereal disease, over 90 percent of Americans said yes.[20] So much for educating Americans on the acceptability of openly discussing syphilis and gonorrhea. Americans were actually *more* progressive on this subject than many in the PHS and the press were.

Parran was undoubtedly well aware that the words *syphilis* and *gonorrhea* were not as taboo as he claimed. During the People's War in which he had played a key role, many of the sex education materials produced by the PHS had used these words. Candid discussions of venereal disease had also been widespread as the government's sex education materials had been posted in community halls, workplaces, and schools. Newspapers had repeatedly used the words *syphilis* and *gonorrhea* rather than common euphemisms when discussing venereal disease throughout the 1910s and 1920s.[21] True, some forms of media, most notably radio, were hesitant to allow the words to be spoken publicly as late as 1936, but in many ways the nation was less reluctant to engage publicly with these words—and more important, with the concept of venereal disease—than public health experts claimed.

Because Parran did not really need to break taboos when he began discussing venereal disease, his actions during this period were probably quite calculated. Parran undoubtedly knew that one of the best ways to launch an aggressive sex education program was through an open discussion of the very words and concepts central to the campaign. Parran also knew that he had greater leeway in speaking publicly about sex and venereal diseases than his counterparts in privately funded organizations; as a representative of the federal government, Parran would not be prosecuted under the Comstock Act for speaking out on the "obscene" topic of sex education.

Mobilizing the Citizen Army

Even before the passage of the National Venereal Diseases Control Act in 1938, the Public Health Service had begun to take steps to revive sex education programs across the nation. State and local boards of health were central to this work, but the PHS also reached out to what Parran and his predecessors called the "citizen army."[22] Once again the PHS tapped community and national organizations to participate. Many of these organizations, such as the General Federation of Women's Clubs and the Rotary Club, had already been involved in the People's War, and they were pleased to be asked to cooperate again. Others, such as the American Social Hygiene Association, had already made the fight against venereal disease their primary mission. These groups were eager to join forces with the Public Health Service again, especially as the PHS made funds more widely available to both these organizations and the communities they served.

Outreach efforts also led the PHS to reinitiate ties with different municipal and religious institutions. Schools became a central battleground for this new campaign, as did churches. The People's War, which had been created with the assistance of the Christian YMCA, had set a strong precedent for working with religious institutions. But the PHS co-opted religious institutions for other reasons. Federal officials believed that the support of the nation's various religious institutions was crucial in quashing opposition from religious groups before it could even emerge. Working closely with churches did, however, have drawbacks, as these partnerships often drove the PHS back into the old practice of equating venereal disease with immorality.

Although the tendency to link venereal disease with immorality was both widespread and deeply rooted in American society, Parran, an extensive traveler, was well aware that not all cultures made this connection. Several Scandinavian countries had created and implemented comprehensive and successful sex education programs that refrained from moral judgments. Parran had been delighted to discover that in Copenhagen "the list of names, places and hours of all venereal disease clinics" was posted alongside "advertisements of department stores, model homes, parks, and other attractions" in the city's main square.[23] Danes suffering from syphilis also had the right to free treatment. In fact, they were legally obligated to submit to this treatment. Parran rather naively believed that Americans could create a similar program. But Denmark was not America; the Danes' long history of pioneering social welfare programs meant that the free medical care Danish syphilitics received rested on policies that were unthinkable in interwar America. Denmark's extraordinarily homogeneous population, which presented a sharp contrast to American society, also ensured that Danish citizens embraced uniform attitudes toward venereal disease. Still, the Danish model could provide an inspiration, and in 1937 Parran translated some Danish policies into American ones. That year he and Raymond Vonderlehr, the director of the Public Health Service's Venereal Disease Division, announced that antisyphilitic drugs would be distributed free of charge and that the PHS would undertake more aggressive epidemiological measures to control syphilis, two efforts that mirrored Danish practices.[24]

States received money from the federal government to fund this new approach. But even before these funds were made widely available, several state and community boards of health had been prepared to take up this battle. Three communities in particular made an early commitment to the fight. Chicago, Baltimore, and New York City all reinstituted the People's War both before and

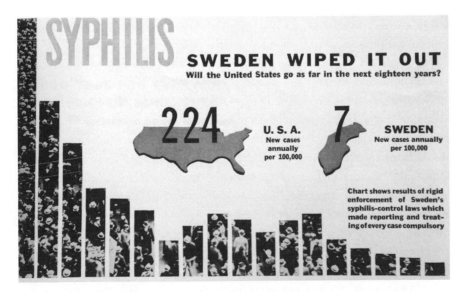

Americans were encouraged to emulate the Scandinavians, who were widely viewed as having the best sex education and venereal disease eradication programs in the world. *Syphilis: Does Your Town Control It?* (1940). Department of Health and Human Services.

as these federal funds were being made available. Working closely with federal officials and public health experts, local authorities and community organizers in these cities took a two-pronged approach to the problem. Educational programs both called for the prevention of venereal disease and encouraged treatment for the infected. In reinvigorating their sex education campaigns, these states looked once again to the federal government. As before, state officials often simply reprinted many of the materials and pamphlets originally produced by the federal government.

Despite the federal government's desire to ensure uniformity in these programs, community-based efforts still reflected regional concerns and stereotypes. This was especially true in regard to efforts to reach African Americans. Unequal access to education, especially in the South, meant that many African Americans lacked basic literacy skills. Not only were many African Americans unable to read sex education pamphlets, they were also more likely to lack access to good health care than their white counterparts. White Americans, many of whom harbored racist views, saw high rates of venereal disease as evidence of African Americans' hypersexuality and natural susceptibility toward disease. African-American reformers, by contrast, emphasized the role racial discrimination had played in fostering high rates of venereal disease among African Americans. In fact, for many middle-class African-American reformers, good sex education was seen as part and parcel of the broader battle for civil rights. For these reformers, a strong bond of racial solidarity made them eager to reach out to their less fortunate peers; unlike white middle-class reformers, who often saw little or no connection between their lives and those of immigrants or working-class whites, African-American reformers tended to be less judgmental and more willing to assess the diverse causes of venereal disease.[25]

In segregated Baltimore, educational efforts incorporated a strong focus on the African-American community. There, a PHS-sponsored survey in 1931 had indicated that venereal disease rates were higher among African Americans than among whites. The survey was developed by white PHS officers, many of whom shared the typically racist views of the day, and it may have provided an inaccurate assessment of the situation. However, the survey did force the Public Health Service to look more closely at public health issues within the often-neglected African-American community. Federal law prohibited African-American physicians from becoming commissioned officers in the PHS, with the result that the PHS and Baltimore city officials were forced to rely on close partnerships with African-American institutions and leaders to promote their sex education initiative in this community. Cooperation with organizations that had participated in the People's War, such as the National Association of Teachers in Colored Schools, ensured that venereal disease exhibits were shown widely in the city's segregated schools.[26] Most African Americans were not, however, in school. To reach these adults, the PHS worked closely with the organizers of National Negro Health Week to promote sex education in the African-American community. Staffed by African-American physicians and professionals, National Negro Health Week was dedicated to improving the health of African Americans. While public health officials in Baltimore were lecturing African Americans on the dangers of promiscuity, the Public Health Service was implementing the Tuskegee Syphilis Experiment. This study, which assessed the effects of untreated syphilis in African-American men, would lead future generations of African Americans to distrust and reject the government's later work to prevent the spread of sexually transmitted diseases in their communities.[27]

Baltimore's prominent white citizens also took up the cause, sometimes to the consternation of local and even federal authorities. Marie Bauernschmidt, the wife of a wealthy brewer, was one of the first to embark on this crusade. Bragging that Baltimore's big "boys . . . have tried to stop me and they have never succeeded," Bauernschmidt had waged a very public war against organized crime and political corruption. Using both her radio show, *Mrs. B. Speaks Her Mind*, and her position as the city's superintendent of schools, Bauernschmidt regularly took on a variety of issues during the 1920s and 1930s.[28]

As a volunteer at the Orthopedic Hospital, Bauernschmidt had confronted the city's seamier side: the "little twisted bodies" of children suffering from the ravages of congenital syphilis. Horrified, Bauernschmidt decided to take the issue public. But speaking out about syphilis proved to be more hazardous than tackling gangsters and corrupt politicians. Despite her strong ties to the city's schools, Bauernschmidt found herself banned from discussing venereal disease in schools. Radio announcers and newspapers forbade her to use the word *syphilis* publicly. Imagine her shock, then, when on a hot summer day she picked up a journal in which the surgeon general of the Public Health Service, Thomas Parran, spoke openly about the dangers of venereal disease and, more surprising still, casually used the word *syphilis*.[29] For Bauernschmidt, the article was an invitation to continue her campaign to educate Baltimoreans on venereal disease.

Now, when school officials banned Bauernschmidt from speaking about sex education, she performed an end run around them by working with the independent Parent-Teacher Association (PTA) to force the issue into the public view. She also took her cause to Congress, testifying publicly about her experiences in promoting sex education.[30] A savvy politician, Bauernschmidt knew that her public testimony before Congress would receive widespread attention. She was also undoubtedly aware of the new shift toward federal intervention in what had previously been seen as local matters. Her fellow Baltimorean H. L. Mencken opted for even more radical measures, demanding that the city's health officials and educators "teach and advocate the use of prophylactic measures" to prevent the spread of venereal disease. Mencken's radical comments, publicized in the *Baltimore Sun*, may have forced some of his fellow citizens to think more creatively about venereal disease.

In addition to prominent Baltimoreans' enthusiasm for the campaign against venereal disease, the city offered other benefits as well. It was home to one of the nation's best medical schools, Johns Hopkins University, and it was close enough to Washington, D.C., to permit frequent cooperation between federal and local authorities.[31] Familiarity brought not contempt but approval. Public Health Service officers were so impressed by Baltimore's campaign that they began indirectly urging cities and states across the nation to follow its model. By the late 1930s and early 1940s, Baltimore's campaign was being replicated across the country.

In New York City, as in Baltimore, public health officials took aggressive action to treat those suffering from venereal disease, even before federal funds were forthcoming. In 1935, New York City boasted one of the best patient-to-clinic ratios in the country. The city's educational program, however, was not quite as impressive. There, the usual culprits—"prudery and an unwillingness to face facts"—were to blame. Further hampering the city's effort was its sprawling size. Because the metropolitan area of New York City included sizable pieces of New Jersey, Connecticut, and even some upstate New York counties, city officials needed to view the venereal disease crisis through a federal, as opposed to state, lens.[32]

By 1936, New York City's public health experts had begun peppering the city with pamphlets and exhibits. Women's clubs and other citizens' organizations held luncheons and evening sessions specifically designed to educate the public about syphilis. Public health officials also noted that the media, especially the *New York Daily News*, had been successfully recruited to help educate the public. In 1939, city officials scored a coup when they piggybacked their program onto the World's Fair. That year, foreign visitors and American nationals who came to New York learned that the "World of Tomorrow" would include better control of syphilis. But the opening of *Scandals*, a "hopped up burlesque show" specifically created to lure World's Fair visitors, suggested that this healthy future was unlikely to begin anytime soon.[33]

There was nothing new in the approach used by New York's Public Health Department. In fact, many of the materials used in this new campaign were recycled from the People's War, and public health officials candidly admitted that they were following "methods similar to those employed in the past." This lack of innovation meant that the program that was instituted would undoubtedly run into many of the same problems that had crippled the People's War fifteen years earlier. But if state and federal authorities failed to develop innovative approaches to public health education, they did call for and ensure that a new emphasis was being placed on sex education in the nation's largest city, which was no mean feat.[34]

In Chicago, officials were no less aggressive than their counterparts in New York City and Baltimore. With great fanfare, officials kicked off a major public health campaign dedicated to eradicating syphilis in 1937. To the relief of the Public Health Service, both municipal and religious authorities embraced the campaign. The city's newspapers, in particular the *Chicago Tribune*, printed "frank, straight-forward facts with regard to venereal disease." Within a few months of the campaign's launch, commuters and workers began finding sex education materials in railroad stations, bus stations, and even the restrooms of their workplaces. The weekends brought no respite from the onslaught as ministers climbed into their pulpits and delivered sermons on the dangers of venereal disease and promiscuity.[35]

Chicago had a long history of working with the Public Health Service to battle venereal disease. During the People's War, many of the PHS's leading consultants had been Chicagoans, and several of these consultants, including Rachelle Yarros, still lived and worked in Chicago in 1937. Yarros had been an enthusiastic supporter of the People's War when it was launched in 1918. Frustrated by what she saw in her own medical practice, Yarros began advocating for the widespread dissemination of birth control information during the 1930s. The Public Health Service officially adopted a much more conservative approach; no PHS official distributed birth control information. For the PHS, concerns about using experts who advocated radical views on sex education were lessened by the belief that these experts brought a wealth of valuable experience to the fight against venereal disease. Besides, the campaign was really focused on the fight against venereal disease. Yarros and other public health experts might believe that women should better understand contraception, but they would have little opportunity to advocate this message when discussing the dangers of syphilis and gonorrhea.[36]

As in New York, public health experts in Chicago used lectures, films, and exhibits in community centers to promote their message. The constant messages had an immediate impact, and the public was quickly roused to action. But as the Public Health Service and Chicago city officials well knew, their tactics were effective only in the short term. Even as the posters began to fade and the lecturers packed their bags and left town, people slipped back into the same dangerous sexual practices.

In the short term, however, the passion that was ignited in Chicago, New York, and Baltimore was shared by other cities. As federal funding became more widely available, neighboring states and communities also took up the cause of sex education. Social Hygiene Day was reinstituted across America. In Greenville, Mississippi, the local paper reminded its readers that local clergymen, schoolteachers, parents, and civic organizations "had done some notable work" in educating residents about the dangers of syphilis. But the work was not yet complete, and local residents were urged to "resolve on this day to continue the work . . . until the prevalence of venereal disease is a fraction of what it is today."[37] Libraries in the heartland risked opposition from local censors by boldly placing the Public Health Service's pamphlets on syphilis and gonorrhea on their shelves and then publicizing the fact in the local newspaper.[38]

Americans have always seen cities as decadent and harboring high rates of venereal disease, but towns, villages, and rural areas have also had their seamy side. In fact, the Public Health Service believed that rates of venereal disease were proportionately higher in rural areas than urban areas. Reaching people in rural areas was difficult, but the PHS saw this as a crucial aspect of the fight against venereal disease. By the late 1930s the PHS was working hard to shake these communities from their complacency by awakening them to the dangers that lurked in even the sleepiest of the nation's towns and villages.[39] In Middletown, New York, the city nurse shocked the Rotary Club by reporting that many students at the local high school were already infected with venereal disease. Urging the teaching of sex education in the city's high school, Nurse Schuerholm sternly reminded her audience that "venereal disease can be wiped out in one generation . . . by means of proper education."[40]

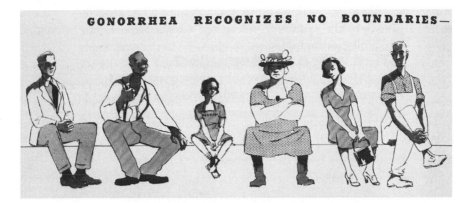

GONORRHEA   RECOGNIZES   NO   BOUNDARIES—

The Public Health Service always emphasized that venereal disease was not limited to any specific subsection of the population. *Twenty Questions on Gonorrhea* (1940). Department of Health and Human Services.

In response to these efforts, requests for educational materials flooded the offices of the Public Health Service. By 1937 the PHS was rushing to meet the demand by supplying state and local authorities with films, posters, exhibits, and pamphlets. Most of these pamphlets and exhibits were simply recycled from the People's War, but increased funding allowed the PHS to begin publishing new pamphlets and producing new films that became available in the late 1930s. The battle lines had clearly been redrawn, and by 1938, PHS officers and public health experts believed, a comprehensive campaign against venereal disease and sexual ignorance could at last be waged—and possibly even be won.

Leaving It to the Experts

Educating adults and communities about the dangers of venereal disease was all well and good, but the PHS had always felt that children and adolescents, especially boys, should be the primary target of any sex education campaign. Many of the Public Health Service's educational materials reflected the hope that parents and ministers would assume the burden of providing sex education. Pamphlets were often directed at making adults, specifically parents, both more comfortable with discussing sex and more knowledgeable about this topic. But as the Service well knew, few parents and even fewer ministers were prepared to provide children with comprehensive sex education. In Maryland, Parran's home state, only 30 percent of the state's adolescents and children had been educated about sex by their parents.[41] Clearly, if sex education was to be taught, the government had no choice but to step in.

Although American children were attending school in record numbers and remaining in school for more years than their parents had, the decentralized nature of the American school system made it impossible to create and implement a standardized sex education program. And yet, as the Public Health Service pointed out, "the schools must . . . assume a major share of the responsibility" for sex education. How could the PHS resolve this dilemma?

In 1939 the Public Health Service began laying the groundwork by publicizing information about a major overhaul of a publication it had issued in partnership with the United States Bureau of Education in 1922. *High Schools and Sex Education* had originally been authored by a PHS consultant, Benjamin Gruenberg. Nearly twenty years later Gruenberg remained active in the field, and he eagerly responded to the Service's request that he rewrite and update his original text by publishing a new edition of the book in 1940.

Reflecting the prejudices of many of his fellow Americans, Gruenberg argued that the recent influx of some 24 million immigrants into America had radically transformed American culture—and not for the better. Gruenberg argued that immigrants' unfamiliarity with traditional American values led them to engage in dangerous sexual practices. Immigrants, he claimed, were behind the rise in venereal disease, illegitimate pregnancy, and even "sex delinquencies." Adding to the problem were the rising divorce rate and the persistence of prostitution, practices that Gruenberg also associated with immigrants. Defined as a "phase of character education," good sex education was cast as a means of Americanizing immigrants and their native-born children by instigating "the socially desirable adult attitudes and practices necessary to insure homemaking [as well as] the establishing and building of families."[42]

Ideally, sex education should be taught as a part of every subject. Along with the biology teacher, teachers in history, English, and even foreign languages should develop lessons designed to provide students with information about sex, sexuality, venereal disease, and the dangers of promiscuity. Teachers who promoted the program needed to be extraordinarily knowledgeable as well as poised and sympathetic. Gruenberg's insistence that teachers also be able to treat the subject humorously while avoiding "dirty" jokes simply complicated the issue. Were there really "clean" jokes about sex?

Implementing such a broad-based program presented several problems.

First, despite everything that the Public Health Service had done with teacher training programs during the 1920s, few teachers were capable of providing the type of comprehensive sex education the PHS advocated. Second, even in those areas where well-trained teachers were available, parental opposition could present serious obstacles. Better teacher education could resolve the first problem, but the second proved more intractable. Gruenberg insisted that "under no circumstances should the principal of a school turn over to any outside individual or organization of parents" the responsibility for sex education. This position undoubtedly reflected the Public Health Service's belief that sex education was best left to the experts—teachers and public health officials.[43]

In a nation that has always been suspicious of "experts," this approach won few supporters. Even public health officials expressed uneasiness with the Public Health Service's view. Thurman Rice, chief of the Bureau of Health and Physical Education of the Indiana Division of Public Health, commended the nation's willingness to teach young people about sex and venereal disease, but he warned against those who wanted schools to provide sex education. Pointing out that most teachers were unmarried, he argued that such "experts" were in fact dangerously ignorant about the realities of sex. Parents, Rice insisted, were best equipped to educate their children on this delicate topic. Citizens who read Rice's comments in the *Hammond Times* had only to look at the article that appeared next to his to know that schools were unable to teach controversial topics; a teacher in Mississippi who disagreed with Darwin had just "ripped an evolution chapter out of his students' textbooks."[44]

Even if Americans had been willing to turn sex education over to public health experts and educators, local authorities' resistance to what they viewed as an encroachment on their authority by the federal government would still have caused problems. No community was willing to allow even indirect federal control over its schools, especially when it came to teaching something as controversial as sex education. In the decades following the publication of Gruenberg's work, parents and "outside organizations" would repeatedly insist that they, not the schools and definitely not the federal government, had the ultimate authority when it came to teaching sex education.[45]

If sex education was contested in the nation's high schools, would it fare any better in the nation's universities? After all, the students at these institutions were adults, at least in a legal sense, and providing them with sex education should be seen as less controversial than providing their younger siblings with the same information.

In 1938, when hearings on the Venereal Disease Control Act were held, college students across the nation had rallied in support of broad sex education initiatives. At Alfred University in New York, students declared that "an enlightened college group can do much to eradicate" venereal disease. In Pennsylvania, students at Moravian College for Women maintained that "a nation invariably looks to its youth for progress . . . [and] straight-forward thinking." There was, college students proclaimed, "no better medium for an active war" against venereal disease than the college newspaper.[46]

College students might be poised to play a significant role in the future as community leaders, educators, doctors, and ministers, but targeting this group with a specially developed sex education campaign would do little to contain venereal disease. Government-sponsored studies had indicated that syphilis rates among college students were lower than among the nation at large. During the 1930s and early 1940s, special sex education programs for college students took a back seat to broader educational efforts.

For the Public Health Service, the promotion of sex education in the nation's schools and colleges would continue to be a major stumbling block in its war on sexual ignorance. Although the PHS repeatedly attempted to shape the structure of sex education programs in schools by providing educators and community leaders with advice and suggestions, it had no real authority to force local communities to follow its guidelines. Limited to encouraging schools to promote sex education by using films and other materials that it provided, the PHS did little to transform the sex education available in American schools during this period.

The federal government's inability to dictate the type of sex education offered in the nation's schools provides some insight into the broader problem of why sex education programs have been so unsuccessful in the United States. In short, if the federal government cannot force schools to use its sex education program, then privately funded sex education programs will be even more ineffective at getting their message across to students in schools.

The More Things Change, the More They . . . Change?

What *was* the message which the Public Health Service was so earnestly attempting to promote in the nation's schools and communities?

As communities began to reinstitute sex education programs during the mid-1930s, the Public Health Service had little new to offer them. Parents and teachers who did contact the PHS for educational materials found themselves receiving dated pamphlets such as *The Parents' Part* and *A Wonderful Story*. The solutions these pamphlets proposed were insufficient to address the intertwined problems of sexual ignorance and venereal disease. Beginning in 1936, improved funding allowed the PHS to produce and release a range of new films, posters, and exhibits. Prominent among these new materials was a series of pamphlets published as Venereal Disease Bulletins. The pamphlets, which sold for approximately 5 cents, were written by the Public Health Service but published and printed under the sponsorship of state boards of health. These bulletins had been a standard component of the People's War.

In 1937 the Public Health Service issued two groundbreaking pamphlets: *Gonorrhea: Its Cause, Its Spread, and Its Cure* and *Syphilis: Its Cause, Its Spread, and Its Cure*. Although other new materials were re-

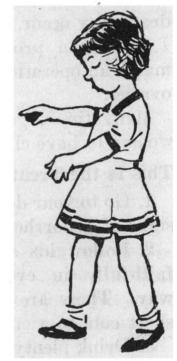

leased at the same time, these two pamphlets would become standards in the Public Health Service's arsenal, remaining in use for several decades. On the surface the pamphlets reiterated the same points that had been made during the People's War. Venereal disease was presented in absolute terms. Gonorrhea, thundered the first of these pamphlets, made men sterile, led women to miscarry, caused heart disease, and, worst of all, infected "little girls . . . who catch it through being handled by a member of the family who has the disease." Syphilis, which caused "thousands of abortions, miscarriages, stillbirths, and syphilitic children," was equally devastating. For those who were immune to these threats, the PHS added a stern warning: insanity, blindness, and heart disease could also be blamed on syphilis.

Because there was nothing new in this bleak assessment of venereal disease, the Public Health Service used strong visuals to drive home its point. Many of these images were updated and recycled from old pamphlets. New and more dramatic images were also used. Seeking to put

The innocent were commonly shown as the victims of syphilis or gonorrhea. *Gonorrhea: Its Cause, Its Spread, and Its Cure* (1937). Department of Health and Human Services.

an end to the old belief that gonorrhea was "a simple disease, like the common cold," the first page of *Gonorrhea: Its Cause, Its Spread, and Its Cure* featured an invalid confined to bed. But it was in *Syphilis: Its Cause, Its Spread, and Its Cure* that the PHS pulled out all the stops. On the first page of the pamphlet, a leering skull and crossbones reminded readers that syphilis caused death.[47]

In these and other pamphlets, the Public Health Service pointed out that syphilis and gonorrhea wrought havoc on the nation's financial well-being. Each year, venereal disease cost the American taxpayer millions of dollars as sufferers failed to contribute to the economy, becoming instead charges on the nation. In Depression-era America, as in Nazi Germany, few taxpayers were willing to support those who had indulged in promiscuous behavior, or even those who were the innocent victims of immoral behavior.[48]

Outside of the financial realm, venereal disease had other, more hidden, costs. During the 1920s, the Public Health Service argued that venereal disease caused racial suicide by rendering its victims sterile. For native-born white Americans who were facing what they regarded as an onslaught on their culture from a massive influx of immigrants, the idea of racial suicide was especially frightening. By the 1930s, with the rise of Nazism, terms such as *racial suicide* and *racial hygiene* had begun to lose their vogue among Americans. Yet even as people became hesitant to use such terms, many native-born white Americans continued to connect the national lack of sex education with the specter of a nation of sickly and degenerate men and women. If a war against venereal disease could eradicate this threat, pouring money into sex education seemed a small price to pay. In fact, pouring money into sex education was the patriotic thing for all Americans to do.[49]

Given these dangers, the question of how to prevent venereal disease remained central to all discussions of sex and sex education. But here the Public Health Service found itself in a quandary. Traditionally public health experts had recommended abstinence as the best means of preventing venereal disease. This approach pleased conservatives, who were easily offended by sex education campaigns that failed to advocate morality. However, as the PHS had discovered during the People's War, aiming low had often meant failing to provide crucial information, information that many Americans genuinely wanted and needed.

Were Americans finally prepared to accept blunt advice that would enable them to avoid venereal disease, even while having sexual intercourse?

In 1937 the Public Health Service decided that the answer to this question was yes. Both *Syphilis: Its Cause, Its Spread, and Its Cure* and *Gonorrhea: Its Cause, Its Spread, and Its Cure* informed readers that "the use of the rubber (condom) during sexual intercourse . . . protects both the man and the woman." In just one short sentence buried at the back of these pamphlets, the PHS had broken the real taboo on discussions of venereal disease.[50] Sex was still pitched as something to be avoided; readers were still warned that even a simple kiss could spread syphilis, and those who were suspected of having venereal disease were still to be shunned, along with any personal objects with which they may have come into contact. But the careful reader would now learn that he or she could have sex and still avoid venereal disease.

There was nothing new or radical in the Public Health Service's promotion of condoms as a means of preventing venereal disease. Since the eighteenth century, Americans and Europeans had used condoms to protect themselves against these diseases. During the 1920s, the introduction of automated technology enabled manufacturers to produce condoms cheaply, quickly, and on an unprecedented scale. As condoms became more readily available, concerns developed regarding their use. In 1930, after a dispute over a patent brought two condom manufacturers into court, the U.S. Court of Appeals for the Second Circuit determined that condoms were illegal when distributed as contraceptives. They were, however, legal when promoted as a means of preventing disease.[51] Translated into practice, this meant that the PHS was free to promote the use of condoms as a means of preventing venereal disease, provided it steered clear of any discussion of their effectiveness in preventing pregnancies. Given the federal government's utter lack of interest in promoting any means of preventing unwanted pregnancies, this decision presented no problems.

The lack of regulations in condom manufacturing did, however, present problems. Throughout the 1910s and 1920s, testing condoms to ensure that they were safe and effective was both expensive and time-consuming. Manufacturers sold "superior" condoms at high prices while selling untested or potentially defective condoms at a cut-rate price. Condom users and their partners were well aware of this practice; when Mary McCarthy lost her virginity as a teenager in 1926, her partner reassured her that the condom was "the *best* kind—a Merry Widow."[52] In 1935, Oregon responded to condom manufacturers' practices by enacting the nation's first law regulating the safety and sale of condoms, and in 1937 the Food and Drug Administration followed suit. These new and comparatively strict federal regulations ensured that Americans were more willing both to trust condoms and to use them.

Despite this new openness regarding condoms, PHS officers undoubtedly held their collective breath following the publication of *Syphilis: Its Cause, Its Spread, and Its Cure* and *Gonorrhea: Its Cause, Its Spread, and Its Cure*. Would there be an outcry condemning the Public Health Service? In 1938 the PHS noted tersely and with great relief that the pamphlets had met with a favorable reaction.[53] The Public Health Service's reluctance to advocate aggressively for the use of condoms undoubtedly forestalled many potential complaints. Parran may have made a great show of saying the word *syphilis* in public, but neither he nor any of the officers under his command publicly discussed in any great detail the information provided in the pamphlets they were now making available to all Americans.

The federal government had taken a dramatic step forward. While the Public Health Service would in years to come often fall back on simple assertions that abstinence was the only real method of avoiding sexually transmitted diseases, the precedent set by these two pamphlets ensured that a growing number of Americans would receive increasingly more comprehensive sex education than their parents had.

CHAPTER FOUR

LIFTING THE SHADOW FROM THE LAND 1941–1945

The people can raze this shadow from the land, from their homes, if the people learn, if they fight syphilis.

FIGHT SYPHILIS, 1942

In peacetime, [venereal disease] lurks like a spider in a dark corner. It rends like a tiger when war comes over the horizon.

SURGEON GENERAL THOMAS PARRAN, 1941

P rostitution is just like any other business," a city official in Washington, D.C., noted with dismay. "It goes where the cash is." During the late 1930s much of the cash came from the unattached young men who had flooded into the nation's capital in the wake of the New Deal. In 1940 the introduction of Selective Service, a peacetime draft, brought a second wave of cash as soldiers and sailors flocked to the city. Within a year it was official: Washington, D.C., home of the federal government and the Public Health Service, had the highest syphilis rates of any city in the nation. Worse yet, prostitutes, eager to accommodate the needs of the market, had begun lowering their prices so that enlisted men could afford their services.[1]

As war threatened, public health officials' concerns escalated. Screening for Selective Service revealed that alarmingly high rates of venereal disease still plagued the nation. What would happen when war began and these men migrated from their home towns to military bases? Would women who left their homes to work in essential war industries become involved in prostitution or, as one North Carolinian newspaper called it, the "girl racket"?[2] And would the "girl racket" cause a spike in rates of venereal disease and illegitimate pregnancies?

The attack on Pearl Harbor on December 7, 1941, followed by the United States' entry into war against Germany, Italy, and Japan, radically altered the federal government's own smaller war on venereal disease and sexual ignorance. In the wake of the war, federally funded sex education programs, both those directed by the Public Health Service and those implemented by other federal institutions, reached record numbers of Americans. In 1941 and then again in 1944, the introduction of new drugs further transformed sex education. Not content to rest on their laurels, federal public health officials used both the introduction of sulfa drugs and penicillin as well as aggressive government initiatives to protect Americans from venereal disease as a foundation for innovative approaches to the control of venereal disease and even illegitimate pregnancies during the postwar period. By the mid-1950s, with rates of venereal diseases declining, the often-repeated claim that these diseases could be "licked" no longer seemed an idle boast. Finally, syphilis and gonorrhea could be relegated to the dust-heap of history.[3]

When the war began, few Public Health Service officers were optimistic about the government's ability to control venereal disease or to limit illegitimate pregnancies. The issue of "military camps and vamps," as one news magazine gleefully called it, had been a serious problem during World War I, and federal officials feared a repeat of this earlier problem. Well aware that chastity and fidelity were typically war's first casualties, congressional legislators, military leaders, and the PHS developed plans to control venereal disease and limit illegitimate pregnancies even before the war began. In 1940 the Senate Committee on Military Affairs held hearings to investigate the causes of these problems. The draft, one witness earnestly explained, "takes boys shortly out of high school, boys who all their lives have been taught to respect women . . . and places them in situations where the absence of normal contact with girls induces a mass lust." Naturally, red-light districts sprang up to cater to this lust. Extensive educational programs and "counter-attractions"—ping-pong, movies, athletics, and a variety of other wholesome activities—were required. But even as they advocated such measures, federal officials knew that a broader and more comprehensive plan was needed.[4]

In 1940 the military, the Public Health Service, and the American Social Hygiene Association (ASHA), a private organization, agreed to cooperate in creating a plan "to defend the armed and industrial forces from venereal disease."[5] Titled the Eight-Point Agreement, this plan called for an expansion of the Service's existing campaign to control venereal diseases. Working together, the Army, Navy, Public Health Service, and ASHA developed and implemented aggressive measures to track the spread of venereal disease, to encourage the infected to seek medical care, to provide treatment to those who were infected, to repress prostitution, and, finally, to promote sex education to arrest the further spread of these diseases. The government benefited from ASHA's expertise in sex education, but ASHA benefited as well. Finally ASHA was able to see, and participate in, the implementation of the broadly based program its leaders had envisioned nearly thirty years earlier. This new approach drew on the diverse powers of the federal government to bolster educational programs with research into the causes and possible treatments for venereal disease, treatment for the infected, and punishment for those who spread the disease.

The forthcoming battle against venereal disease was now "fundamental to the defense aims of this country," and Surgeon General Parran took the campaign seriously—so seriously that he was willing to jeopardize his career by launching a public attack on military leaders who he believed had refused to step up to the plate.[6] In 1941, shortly before the war began, Parran published his second bestseller, *Plain Words about Venereal Disease*, in which he charged military leaders with complacency in the face of the venereal disease threat. The Army, Parran alleged, was especially negligent in preparing for and fighting the war against sexual ignorance. This very public criticism of the military's lackadaisical approach received widespread attention, enraging Parran's boss, President Franklin D. Roosevelt. "If the Surgeon General of the Army or the Surgeon General of the Navy had written this book . . . he would have been liable to court martial," fumed Roosevelt.[7] But Parran's critique earned high praise in communities ranging from Cumberland, Maryland, to Brownsville, Texas.[8] With or without help from the federal government, these communities were prepared to fight and conquer venereal disease and sexual ignorance.

Finding the Enemy

On a visit to Washington, D.C., a country practitioner stopped by the offices of the Public Health Service. "Folks down my way sure got het up about syphilis when they read all about it in the magazines," he told Surgeon General Parran. Patients had "come a-flockin' to find did they have [the disease]." Here was the proof Parran needed. Newspaper articles, poster exhibits, films, and open discussions about syphilis—sex education—could change people's behavior, encouraging them to be checked and treated for venereal disease.[9]

In Lumberton, North Carolina, citizens agreed with Parran's assessment of the power of sex education. Two months after the war had begun, the town prepared to celebrate Social Hygiene Day. The local health department vowed that "no discovered case of syphilis should remain untreated at large in the community to infect others," but the Robison County Health Department could not wage this war alone. Venereal disease eradication is a " 'home front' job for every town in the United States," the local paper reminded its residents. Individual citizens, community organizations, schools, and churches all needed to join the fight.[10]

Because America's soldiers, sailors, and industrial workers came from the full range of the nation's cities, towns, and farms, screening for the draft provided a comprehensive snapshot of the nation's venereal disease crisis. As doctors found case after case, national patterns of gonorrhea and syphilis rates became evident on a state-by-state basis. The nation's highest disease rates were in Mississippi, home to Dr. Felix Underwood, who had testified so movingly on the ravages of syphilis in 1938. Horrified, state officials leaped to point the finger at African Americans, claiming that "Negro syphilitics . . . don't think being cured [of syphilis] is worth it."[11] According to these and other white officials, African Americans were not only less inclined to seek treatment, they were also *more* inclined to become infected than whites. To explain these higher rates of infection, many whites pointed to what they claimed was African Americans' hypersexuality. However, more enlightened public health experts in the Public Health Service, the military, and African-American organizations such as the National Medical Association knew the real cause for these higher rates: poverty, poor education, and limited access to medical care. In short, socioeconomic factors, not race, were central in determining both why people became infected and how they responded to the condition.

No one race, class, or gender had a monopoly on venereal disease; even the most racist state and local public health officials acknowledged that venereal disease cut across race, class, and gender lines. But although public health officials conceded that venereal disease could be found in every segment of American society, they also knew that the poor, as well as the less educated, were more inclined to become infected with venereal disease (the poor were also more likely to suffer from other diseases such as ringworm, pellagra, and even tuberculosis). In segregated America, African Americans disproportionately lived in poverty. Compared with whites, the majority of African Americans had limited or no real access to educational opportunities, good wages, or health care, all factors that were crucial in protecting Americans from venereal disease and ensuring that those who were infected received treatment. At the start of the war, African Americans still overwhelmingly lived in rural poverty across the South. Living within the boundaries of the former Confederacy meant that they also lived within a segregated society that denied them both a good education and readily available health care. Compounding these problems was the widespread practice of sharecropping, which had placed extraordinary pressures on the African-American family. By 1940 these pressures had created a situation in which "sexually transmitted diseases . . . were nationally known as special problems of the black rural South."[12] Given this situation, the need for sex education programs was especially crucial in the South. But in Mississippi, as elsewhere in the South, conservative upper-class white officials saw little or no need to provide programs that they believed benefited African Americans or even poor whites. As long as segregation remained a central component of Southern culture—and America continued to be segregated even as African-, Asian-, and Native-American soldiers fought for democracy abroad—federal funds were desperately needed simply to ensure that sex programs could reach those who needed them. Both immediately before and during the war, these federal funds transformed the battle against sexual ignorance and the problems caused by this ignorance throughout the United States but especially in the South by ensuring that all races and classes received some form of sex education.

The prejudices expressed in Mississippi were not unique to the South; even in places as far north as Madison, Wisconsin, the belief that African Americans were somehow to blame for the nation's high rates of syphilis was repeatedly emphasized in the local papers.[13] African-American leaders had long called upon the Public Health Service to include and allocate funding for their communities when planning public health initiatives. Pointing out that African Americans had responded positively to many such federally funded initiatives, African-American leaders saw an opportunity in this new push for better sex education. Close cooperation with the PHS brought well-funded public health initiatives into their communities. But these initiatives proved to be a double-edged sword. The racism that led to the Public Health Service's enthusiasm for this initiative also ensured the continuation of not only the Tuskegee Syphilis Experiment and racist views of sexuality but also the belief that African Americans were like children, unable to care for themselves.

Amid all this finger-pointing, public health officials did not lose sight of the big picture, and they increasingly began to emphasize what had long been their mantra: venereal disease cut across lines of race, class, and gender. If nothing else, the war, which took teenagers and young adults away from their families and then turned them into soldiers and sailors who were exposed to all sorts of temptations, proved that no one was safe from the threat of venereal disease. To reach these Americans, as well as their sisters and sweethearts, public health officials now insisted that the war on venereal disease entail a multifaceted approach, one that was possible only through the diverse agencies of the federal government.

Does Your Town Control Venereal Disease?

With the outbreak of war, San Francisco officially became a part of the western theater. A major port, the city had always had its share of vice, but now, with the influx of soldiers and sailors, its seamier side was revealed to all Americans. Jean, a young teenager, experienced that vice firsthand. Unmarried and pregnant at seventeen, she induced an abortion. Within a year she was pregnant again. This time she gave birth to an illegitimate child. To save face, her mother told their neighbors that Jean had married and her husband was stationed overseas. Although Jean was not suffering from venereal disease and although she did not engage in prostitution, her future, at least according to public health experts, looked bleak. Studies indicated that 80 percent of women like Jean contracted venereal disease. As reservoirs of disease, these women were doomed to a shortened life of ill-health. True, some "promiscuous" women would *not* contract venereal disease, but even for these women there were dangers. At best, illegitimate pregnancies and a life on relief were in their future. At worst, death from a botched abortion in a dark alleyway loomed. More worrisome still, the sexual misbehavior of Jean and women like her put men and their innocent wives at risk of contracting venereal disease.[14]

The advent of the war caused prostitutes and "good time girls" to swarm into cities and towns with essential war industries or military camps. Newspapers and city officials reported "a sharp increase in girls' sex delinquencies."[15] In Dallas, parents were warned that their daughters might be in a "downtown tavern giving come-hither smiles to soldiers and acquiring and spreading venereal disease."[16] In Reno, officials may have preferred to believe that rumors claiming that the majority of girls in the city suffered from venereal disease were "mean-spirited [and] malicious" and gave "aid and comfort to the enemy," but the city's high rates of venereal disease indicated that the rumors probably had some basis in fact.[17] No city was immune. Even New York City, which had launched a

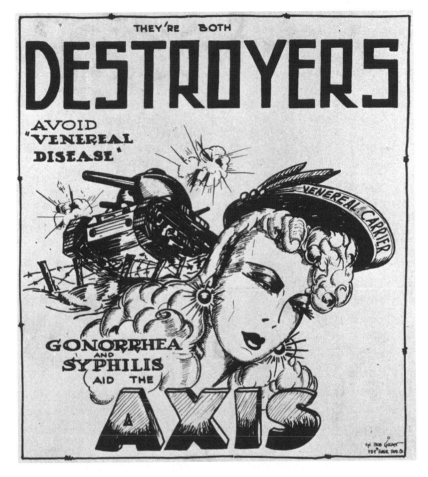

Women like Jean were as dangerous as the soldiers and weapons of the Axis (ca. 1940s).
Department of Health and Human Services.

model sex education initiative in the 1930s, saw its juvenile delinquency rate
double. Many of the underage girls who appeared in the city's courts were "pregnant and a still larger number [had] syphilis or gonorrhea."[18] By January 1943,
two years after the war began, the New York City Health Department reported
a "20% rise in venereal disease rates among adolescents, both boys and girls."[19]

Clearly, drastic measures were needed. City officials in Waco, Texas, took a
typically hard line, imposing a curfew and sending teenagers home after 5 P.M.
in an attempt "to curb the spread of venereal diseases."[20] Prostitutes, whether

teenagers or older women, were arrested and forced to undergo treatment if they were infected with venereal diseases. In this climate, calls for "social control" rooted in sex education took on a new urgency.[21] As Americans increasingly acknowledged the importance of sex education, communities throughout the country found themselves amid one of the most extensive public health campaigns the federal government had ever launched.[22] More posters, more pamphlets, more films, and more books poured out from the Public Health Service's Venereal Disease Division. Across the United States, communities rallied, presenting talks and exhibits on venereal disease that used these sex education materials.

At the heart of this campaign were private-public partnerships. The federal government aggressively funded private organizations, providing them with grants and assistance in creating materials that could be distributed both nationally and locally. In North Carolina, the VD Education Institute, which had been founded in 1931 with money from the tobacco heir Smith Reynolds, received substantial federal funds during the war. Using these funds, the institute developed and distributed materials to educate the "average person" about venereal disease.[23] Organizations such as the VD Education Institute provided a good return on the federal dollar, as they typically matched federal funds with their own money. Programs created by these private organizations also had the added benefit of not appearing to come from the federal government. Citizens who were concerned about "federal meddling" in sex education often did not know or understand that these privately produced materials were made possible through their taxpayer dollars. As a result, these programs did not encounter much opposition. As had been true with many of their older partnerships, these new initiatives allowed the federal government to dictate the shape of an extraordinary number of sex education initiatives in the United States, even programs that appeared to be independent of the federal government.

The sex education programs that emerged during the war also continued to rely on the same formal and informal partnerships with private and more broadly based organizations that had characterized earlier sex education campaigns. The General Federation of Women's Clubs, for example, once again took up the cause of sex education. GFWC members worked, as they had previously, to arrange lectures, films, and exhibits designed to provide sex education. Similarly, the YMCA, Rotary Clubs, and other locally based organizations also received support and funding from the Public Health Service to promote sex education.

However, the Public Health Service was not content simply to rely on organizations with which they had an established relationship. Federal officials also actively sought out new organizations and new means to promote sex education. Among these new partners was the Ad Council, an association of advertisers formed in the early 1940s to foster a positive image of advertising by promoting social and patriotic causes. After 1942 the renamed War Advertising Council developed highly successful propaganda campaigns for the federal government, including the iconic campaign featuring Rosie the Riveter. But when the War Advertising Council worked with the PHS to develop a morally neutral sex education campaign, they ran into trouble. Catholic organizations believed that the teaching of morality was integral to sex education, and the New York branch of the Knights of Columbus angrily told Surgeon General Parran that a morally neutral "advertising campaign is certainly not the proper medium" to eradicate venereal disease. Sex education, the Knights of Columbus insisted, should begin and end with "the private counsel of the parent, the teacher or the spiritual advisor"—not with a public ad campaign. A Catholic himself, Parran agreed that parents and clergymen should teach morality, but he also believed that morality was fundamentally irrelevant to public health education. Parran argued, instead, that good sex education—which was, after all, a form of health education—should emphasize the "medical and public health aspects of venereal disease control." Catholic organizations disagreed, and during the fall of 1944 the Knights of Columbus, Catholic clergymen, the Catholic media, and other organizations launched their own war on the government's campaign. Concerned that this opposition from Catholic consumers would threaten the advertising business overall, the War Advertising Council suspended its cooperation with the Public Health Service in 1944.[24]

This joint effort with the War Advertising Council was a rare failure. More successful was the Public Health Service's use of Hollywood to develop and promote sex education films intended for civilians. Like the War Advertising Council, the Research Council of the Academy of Motion Picture Arts became heavily involved in the war effort. During the war the Research Council conducted courses for Signal Corps officers and ran schools for Signal and Marine Corps cameramen. The Council also broke new ground in sex education films when it developed *Know for Sure*, a sex education film it produced for the Public Health Service. Released in 1941, *Know for Sure* was aimed at male workers in wartime industries. The film used several well-known actors, including Hattie McDaniel, the African-American actress who had so recently won an Oscar for her performance in the wildly popular film *Gone with the Wind. Know for Sure* followed a plot line familiar to those who had seen Upton Sinclair's play *Damaged Goods* or read Nancy Hale's story "The Blue-Muslin Sepulchre": after the birth of his child, a father discovers that he has passed syphilis on to the infant. Although the plot line was tired, the film's creators did break new ground by promoting and candidly discussing the use of prophylaxis in preventing venereal disease. This promotion of prophylaxis was seen as so controversial that the government's major private partner, ASHA, protested the use of this film. State officials, such as the director of the Montana State Board of Health, were even more vocal in denouncing the film, arguing that it opened a door to "sexual immorality and birth control." But Raymond Vonderlehr, the director of the Public Health Service's Venereal Disease Division, saw the situation quite differently. "Teaching men how to protect themselves from venereal disease does not," Vonderlehr argued, "imply that we condone sexual promiscuity no more than teaching soldiers how to protect themselves against poison gas proves that the Army wishes to encourage the use of such gas by the enemy." Vonderlehr's justification was almost unnecessary, as *Know for Sure* was extraordinarily well received by filmgoers across the country, and the film quickly became a staple in sex education programs directed at both civilians and military recruits.[25]

Overall the Public Health Service's wartime partnerships with organizations such as the Academy of Motion Picture Arts tended to be extremely successful, reaching millions of Americans and educating them on the dangers of venereal disease. In some ways the success of these efforts stemmed from the widespread belief that volunteerism was central to the American way of life. But many Americans also genuinely believed that private organizations could and should perform tasks that in other countries were governmental responsibilities. During the war, patriotism spurred these citizens to devote more of their time and efforts to a variety of public initiatives, including sex education.[26] In the past, communities had always responded to federally funded sex education campaigns with a great deal of enthusiasm, especially in the early years of these campaigns, but the war brought a new sense of urgency to the battle against sexual ignorance. When mandatory screening for Selective Service and the draft revealed high levels of venereal disease, communities were finally forced to acknowledge that the problem existed in their own backyards. The threat posed by the war also provided Americans with a new and very dramatic understanding of the Public Health Service's oft repeated claim that controlling venereal disease was central to the nation's defense and its very survival.

Educators Must Aid in Cutting through False Modesty

War put extreme pressures on the American family. Some of these pressures were external, as when fathers and sons were drafted and sent overseas or when mothers and fathers moved families to take jobs in wartime industries. But other pressures were less easy to define and reflected Americans' general uneasiness with the changes that were occurring in their own society. As has always been true in times of national stress, Americans felt themselves to be overwhelmed by rebellious teenagers. Adults had only to pick up the newspaper to see how American society was under attack by these immoral teens. In one story about a fifteen-year-old girl who had run away from her home in Texas, the decline of American morals was evident even to the most cursory of readers. Appalled social workers had discovered the young girl in a hotel "alone, undressed in bed. On the dresser were twenty-three beer bottles . . . and two empty pint bottles of whiskey and one pint of rum half gone." The runaway greeted the social workers by cheerfully informing them that she had been entertaining sailors in her room. Had the social workers arrived just thirty minutes earlier, she bragged, they "would have walked in on a party of five sailors and two other girls."

This teenager may have simply been looking to shock her listeners, but her story and similar ones were seen as evidence of deeper problems in American society. From the zoot suit riots in Los Angeles to the rising violence of teens in Dallas, Americans believed, incorrectly, that juvenile delinquency was reaching new levels.[27] Arguing that "young girls . . . often copy the behavior of older ones," some Americans insisted that the sheer prevalence of prostitutes and good-time girls encouraged teenagers to adopt their elders' wild behavior. Still others insisted that adolescents' rebellious behavior stemmed from the "breaking up of homes during the war, the moving of residences because of war industrial work and the failure of communities to provide adequate recreational facilities."[28]

Faced with a barrage of stories highlighting teenagers' bad behavior, Americans overwhelmingly agreed that schools should provide sex education. By 1943 the percentage of Americans advocating school-sponsored sex education significantly outweighed those who opposed it: 66 percent of men and 69 percent of women were in favor of these courses. Community organizations also demanded that school districts implement sex education classes. In 1942, for example, 2.5 million club women publicly advocated "a sex education program for adolescents, to be provided with the aid of school authorities." Similarly, the

American Social Hygiene Association, which had partnered with the Public Health Service to promote sex education, insisted that "educators . . . must aid in cutting through the false modesty and taboos connected with venereal disease." Support for sex education was greatest in urban areas and the North, but support was also high in the nation's farming communities and the South, and all of these communities rallied to support this initiative.[29]

Calls to implement sex education courses in high schools came at an opportune time. In earlier decades the Public Health Service had struggled to reach teenagers who could be found both in schools and the workforce. During the 1930s, school enrollments soared as more adolescents remained in school for longer periods. The war saw a slight dip in the percentage of adolescents who were in school as many male students enlisted and both male and female students joined the workforce. But even this slight decline did not hide the fact that three-quarters of all teenagers between the ages of fourteen and seventeen were now enrolled in school.[30] Finally, programs developed for schools would enable the Public Health Service to reach the majority of the nation's adolescents. Other, broader changes in the structure of the American high school also provided opportunities to promote sex education. Patriotic fervor made many schools especially receptive to the goals of military and federal agencies, enabling locally based PHS officials to speak more directly to administrators and school boards. Additionally, because screening for the draft had revealed that many of the nation's young men were physically unfit for service, schools developed new, or in some instances more comprehensive, physical education programs. Health education, which often fell under the aegis of physical education programs, benefited from this expansion of the high school curricula.[31]

But even as high schools demonstrated a new receptiveness toward sex education, the key question remained: What kind of sex education should the schools provide?

Public Health Service officials had attempted to address this question in 1940 when they asked Benjamin C. Gruenberg to update his book *High Schools and Sex Education*. The publication of Gruenberg's work had been widely trumpeted in the press, but the decentralized nature of the American school system meant that educators' willingness to read and incorporate Gruenberg's work varied from district to district. Problems that had existed before the war—poor teacher training and limited access to PHS materials—continued to plague those schools districts that attempted to implement Gruenberg's suggestions.

The war, which caused teacher shortages and overcrowding, simply exacerbated these existing problems. Yet even as these problems emerged, some school districts began promoting sex education quite aggressively. In Dallas, where the Parent-Teacher Association was "100 per cent behind the new [sex education] program," administrators and physical education teachers worked with parents to implement a comprehensive new program.[32]

The Public Health Service was eager to have other communities follow the lead set by Dallas and other cities. In 1944 the PHS attempted once again to address this issue by assigning one of its officers, Dr. Lester Kirkendall, to work with the Department of Education to promote sex education in the schools. Although the Department of Education had only limited powers to control and direct the nation's schools, its ability to shape the nation's curricula was greater than that of the Public Health Service.

"It's ostrich like to think our young people are not informed [about] . . . sex unless we choose to tell them," Kirkendall lectured his fellow Americans. The war had swept away all inhibitions, ensuring that sex was "already treated openly in books, newspapers, movies, and conversations."[33] But even as he preached a new openness toward sex education, Kirkendall's approach remained, at heart, deeply conservative. The Public Health Service's studies seemed to indicate that a knowledge of prophylaxis encouraged teenagers to engage in sexual experimentation. While the studies the PHS had conducted were, by modern standards, flawed, Kirkendall believed their results, and he refused to teach adolescents about condoms. This refusal, combined with concerns that "youngsters may take a flippant attitude" toward sex education, led the PHS to advocate courses "aimed at the improvement of human relations and the strengthening of family life." Despite Parran's insistence that the PHS would leave the teaching of morals to parents and clergymen, Kirkendall and the Department of Education wound up advocating that the nation's schools teach sexual morality in place of public health education.[34] But even as Kirkendall violated Parran's views on health education, his approach reflected broader cultural trends. Stories about drunken fifteen-year-olds entertaining sailors in hotel rooms and teenagers roaming the streets were probably often exaggerated and did not reflect the very real decline in crime that occurred during the war. They did, however, clearly reflect Americans' fears about the state of their nation. Threatened from without, Americans were eager for sex education programs that would reassure them that their society was not shifting from within.

Camps and Vamps

Pastor Norbert Talbot took both his patriotism and his religious duties seriously. In 1943 he left his church in Huntingsburg, Indiana, and, along with some 2,900 other ministers, entered the Naval Training School for Chaplains in Williamsburg, Virginia. After Talbot completed his training, a naval board asked him how he would respond when his commanding officer demanded that he educate sailors on venereal disease and prophylaxis. "Bowled over" by the question, Talbot retorted that his religious beliefs prevented him from carrying out such orders. The Navy quickly released Talbot from military duty.[35]

Having lost over 7.5 million working days to venereal disease during World War I, the American military was determined that this new war would be different. If protecting the nation's 16 million male recruits—and its 350,000 female recruits—from venereal disease meant providing them with information about prophylaxis, both the Army and the Navy were now prepared to do so. In fact, even before the war had begun the military had assumed that sailors and soldiers did not practice abstinence and provided them with information about condoms. The Public Health Service, which served the Merchant Marines, had made a similar assumption about the sailors under its own watch; in the 1920s, pamphlets such as *Whither Away?* used frank language and provided merchant seamen with detailed information on how to protect themselves against venereal disease.

Educating draftees about the dangers of illicit sexual intercourse and the benefits of preventive measures when engaging in this behavior would be easier than educating civilians. The decentralized structure of the American school system had always made it difficult for federal officials to create and mandate a uniform sex education program. But now, as the federal government mobilized the nation's men, there was a unique opportunity to present citizens in the armed forces with a uniform and mandatory sex education program. Equally important, the war finally enabled government officials to direct and implement a sex education program that would be relatively free of interference from parents, ministers, and teachers. Communities often varied in their implementation of this program, and private organizations such as the American Social Hygiene Association did participate in the military's campaign, but this remained very much the government's program.

The government left nothing to chance. Sex education was viewed as so important that it began with induction into the military. Chaplains such as Pastor

Norris, along with military officers, were expected to give soldiers and sailors a talk on venereal disease almost immediately upon their reporting for duty. Additional programs on venereal disease then followed at regular intervals. Cartoons, films, posters, and pamphlets all provided soldiers and sailors with detailed information about the dangers of promiscuity.[36] Stoking recruits' fear of venereal disease was the dominant theme of these programs. Recruits were repeatedly reminded of the consequences of venereal disease: over and over the government stressed that venereal disease caused lasting damage to one's health, fertility, sexual capacity, and family life. Fear was believed to be a highly effective deterrent, although military leaders were prepared to use other tactics. Appeals to morality were also common, but even as they advocated continence as the "moral" approach to sexual matters, military leaders and public health experts recognized that these appeals were "of limited value."[37]

Looking back at the government's message in later years, many soldiers and sailors characterized it as simply "KPIP," or "Keep Pecker in Pocket."[38] But the government's message was actually more nuanced than that. Recognizing that "angels rightfully only belong in heaven," the military and the Public Health Service took active steps to ensure that soldiers and sailors learned about the effectiveness of condoms in preventing the spread of venereal disease. Better still, after learning about condoms, draftees could easily obtain them from shops and even vending machines. And obtain them they did. During the war about 50 million condoms were distributed on a monthly basis to the troops.[39]

This approach came under scrutiny despite the fact that the military and the Public Health Service trod lightly when speaking about and advocating new sex education programs that included frank discussions of condoms. In 1941, as huge numbers of men were drafted or enlisted in the Army and Navy, military leaders were attacked both for their approach to sex education and for their willingness to provide soldiers and sailors with condoms. For those in the military who were the object of the public's anger, lowered rates of venereal disease over the course of the war must have provided some comfort.

Much more popular was the federal government's hard-line approach to the camp followers who traditionally flocked to military bases. The May Act, which was passed in 1941, enabled the Justice Department to override local authorities and directly police areas that presented a threat to the safety of either military or industrial workers. Venereal disease was regarded as a major threat to the well-being of the American military, and Eliot Ness, who had made his reputation fighting bootleggers like Al Capone, now turned his attention to a dif-

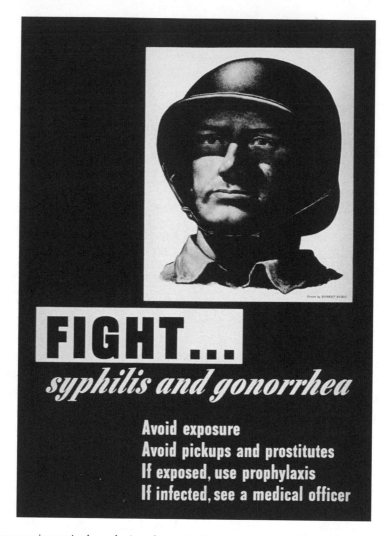

FIGHT...

syphilis and gonorrhea

Avoid exposure
Avoid pickups and prostitutes
If exposed, use prophylaxis
If infected, see a medical officer

Military recruits received very basic and very simple instructions on dealing with venereal disease (ca. 1940s). Department of Health and Human Services.

ferent type of vice. Under Ness' guidance, federal officials launched a full-scale war on the prostitutes and "good-time girls" who serviced military bases and industrial centers. Directing the Social Protection Division under the Office of Community War Services, Ness and his "untouchable" crime-fighters became the government's key front men in the war against prostitution and its corollary, the war against venereal disease. Widely discussed in both the civilian and military press, the very public clean-up campaign that Ness directed did as much to educate soldiers, sailors, and communities near military bases on the dangers of unregulated sex as the government's more official campaign.

Does She Look Clean? Know for Sure

Moviegoers across the United States watched with patriotic pride as soldiers strutted across the screen in perfect formation. As the parade passed, a veteran of World War I turned his back on the soldiers and was assisted into a wheelchair. A war wound? No, this soldier had been felled by the real enemy: syphilis.[40]

By 1941 many of the sex education materials that the Public Health Service had begun developing during the late 1930s were finally available. PHS films such as *Know for Sure* and *Fight Syphilis* took center stage in this campaign. *Know for Sure*, a "Hollywood produced motion picture that pulls no punches but shows men exactly how to 'play safe' and what to do to escape syphilis," was released in 1942. "The latest shot fired by the United States Public Health Service in its war on syphilis," the film was originally intended to "be shown only to men's groups in clubs, factories, colleges, and possibly army training camps."[41] Other films, such as *Fight Syphilis, Personal Hygiene for Men*, and *Personal Hygiene for Women*, were also released. By 1945 the PHS was noting with some satisfaction that six "dramatic radio programs" about venereal disease had been produced in Hollywood. These were made available for wider distribution by the nation's various state and local health departments. Better yet, a new Technicolor sex education film intended for women and girls was in the works.[42]

Along with these films and radio shows, the Public Health Service also released a series of new pamphlets designed to educate Americans about the threat facing their communities. Some of these pamphlets, such as *Twenty Questions on Gonorrhea* and *Syphilis: Does Your Town Control It?* had been written and released before the war. But others such as *Victory vs. VD* were new and specifically tailored to the war effort. In 1937 two PHS pamphlets, *Syphilis: Its Cause, Its Spread, and Its Cure* and *Gonorrhea: Its Cause, Its Spread, and Its Cure*, had told Americans that condoms would protect them against venereal disease. The publication of these pamphlets had provoked no real outcry, and during the war both continued to be available to those who requested them. But PHS officials had always viewed these pamphlets with some trepidation, and they did not promote this message widely either before or during the war. Between 1941 and 1957, new pamphlets intended for civilians overwhelmingly sidestepped the issue of condoms. Instead, they focused on mobilizing communities to deal with venereal disease through calls for legislation requiring blood tests at the time of marriage, the creation of free clinics, and even free testing for citizens who were not preparing to be married. Although effective, these new educational materials provided Americans with only half the information they needed to prevent the spread of venereal disease in their communities.

If these pamphlets, films, and radio shows failed to educate Americans about how to fully protect themselves from venereal disease and illegitimate pregnancies, what did these materials tell Americans about venereal disease and those who contracted it?

Syphilis, Americans were told, began in the "dangerous" parts of cities, with "easy pick-ups" on "dark hidden streets." Just one encounter with a syphilitic woman, and a chain of infection could spread outward, infecting even the "safe" areas of a city.[43] Promiscuous women, the government warned, spread disease, infecting healthy men and hampering the war effort. Yet even as the government's educational propagandists made this claim, federal officials were admitting, at least privately, that many of these women were themselves the victims of poor sex education.

Blaming girls like Jean, the "immoral" young woman in San Francisco, for the spread of venereal disease stemmed, no doubt, from the government's concerns that soldiers, sailors, and workers needed to be protected if the war was to be won. But this focus led, at best, to a slanted view of sexuality and sexual mores as women were once again divided into two types: the good girl and the girl "who looked clean" but was not. Worse yet, this view did little to protect women who engaged in extramarital intercourse. But because many of these women worked in essential industries, this approach also threatened the broader war effort.

Despite these problems, the appeal of this type of campaign was obvious. It was easy to understand and implement. Additionally, by linking immorality and venereal disease, this campaign would please even the most conservative members of American society, thereby ensuring that Americans overwhelmingly supported it. But federal officials also advocated this approach because they believed it to be highly effective. If encouraging men to believe that women who engaged in sexual intercourse outside of marriage were all diseased prevented these men from engaging in risky behavior, then the program would be a success. Similarly, if encouraging women to believe that engaging in extramarital sexual intercourse would mark them as "bad" women, then women could also be prevented from engaging in risky behavior.

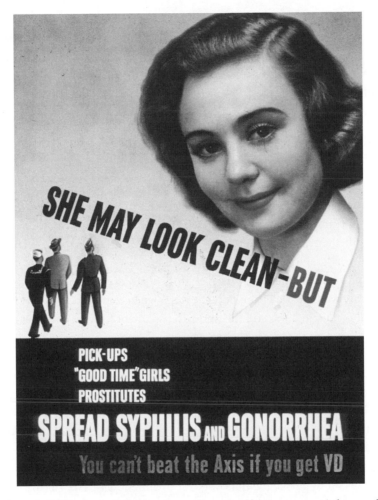

SHE MAY LOOK CLEAN – BUT

PICK-UPS
"GOOD TIME" GIRLS
PROSTITUTES
SPREAD SYPHILIS ᴀɴᴅ GONORRHEA
You can't beat the Axis if you get VD

In the absence of a blood test, there was no way of knowing if this woman carried venereal disease (ca. 1940s). Department of Health and Human Services.

There was one small flaw with this approach. Repeated studies had demonstrated that fear was often overridden by desire: fear was not, in other words, an effective deterrent in the long term. At a loss as to how to address this problem, the Public Health Service fell back on its old tactic of simply flooding communities with pamphlets, films, and posters. And yet even as they followed this old and problematic tactic, the Public Health Service and the federal government noted that their war on sexual ignorance and venereal disease was also moving smoothly toward victory. Rates of venereal disease were down among civilians.

Rates of illegitimate pregnancies were still high, but this issue had never really been the focus of the government's campaign. For the Public Health Service, the educational effort had finally begun to "raze the shadow [of venereal disease] from the land"—just as foretold in 1942.[44]

Or had it?

Rapid Treatments

In 1942, newspapers reported that the Army was accepting into its ranks men who were suffering from venereal disease. After being accepted, these men, all of whom were suffering from uncomplicated cases of gonorrhea, were treated and cured with a new drug, sulfathiozel. "Cured by the draft," these men could now fulfill their patriotic duty, and as the nation geared up for war, Parran boasted that "gonorrhea now can be wiped out."[45]

Curing syphilis remained, however, difficult to do, and men suffering from this disease were excused from duty. In 1941, when the war began, Salvarsan, an arsenical compound, was still the standard treatment for venereal disease. Since its discovery in the early twentieth century, Salvarsan had been heralded as a "magic bullet." But Salvarsan had problems. Unlike a simple antibiotic, it was administered by intravenous injection, a procedure that required the patient to visit a physician.[46] Worse yet, to be effective the drug needed to be administered over a prolonged period of time, requiring a serious commitment on the part of the patient. If all this was not enough to deter a patient, then the exorbitant price of the drug would certainly give sufferers pause, especially in a nation that lacked widely available health care insurance. No surprise, then, that many patients were reluctant to pursue the full course of treatment necessary to cure syphilis.

Because Salvarsan provided the only effective means of treating syphilis at this time, the Public Health Service had little choice but to promote its use. This promotion took several forms. The most famous of these was a film that the PHS co-produced with Warner Brothers shortly before the outbreak of World War II. Clearly intended as a back-door form of sex education, *Dr. Ehrlich's Magic Bullet* starred Edward G. Robinson as Paul Ehrlich, the discoverer of Salvarsan. Robinson, who had made a career of playing tough gangsters, now took on and defeated two real thugs: syphilis and public prudery. But even Robinson's popularity was unable to cure Americans of their suspicions about the drug.

All this changed with the introduction of penicillin in 1944. Now a simple course of antibiotics could cure syphilis.

Even before penicillin became available, the government had taken aggressive measures to contain and control venereal diseases. In 1941 the government had recognized that the creation and expansion of military bases as well as the growth of wartime industries had led to a massive population shift as Americans flocked to new jobs or enlisted in the military. Local taxpayers, who funded the schools and services that served these new transients, found themselves struggling to assume the financial burden that came with this migration. In 1941 Congress passed the Lanham Act, which was designed to ease the local tax burden by providing communities with federal funds that could be used to build and support community facilities. The Act specifically provided funds for hospitals where carriers of venereal disease could be quarantined until they had been cured. Throughout the war, as federal dollars poured into local communities, venereal disease hospitals were opened across the country. Funded by the federal government but operated by state and local authorities, these "rapid treatment" centers "provide[d] care for prostitutes and other promiscuous females who have a venereal disease."[47] Definitions of prostitution and promiscuity proved, however, to be trickier to establish than hospitals. As the war progressed, it became clear that "prostitutes" or "promiscuous females" were often women who were simply guilty of living lives that did not fit most Americans' narrow definition of a woman's role. In Rapid City, South Dakota, for example, women who were "continually on the streets and whose behavior seem[ed] questionable" could be detained on suspicion of spreading venereal disease. They could then be subjected to detention within a clinic.[48] By 1946, as soldiers and sailors were being demobilized, nearly one-third of all cases of syphilis that were reported to state health departments were being treated and cured in these "rapid-treatment" centers.[49]

This extraordinary measure—in which the government deprived "promiscuous" women of their rights by detaining them and then forcing them to undergo treatment for venereal disease—was, the Public Health Service, claimed, a highly effective tool for controlling venereal disease. But the situation was more complex than the government admitted. While diseased women were forced to undergo treatment, "diseased men declared ineligible for the draft returned to their communities where, in many cases, no treatment was provided."[50] Across America, even as rates of venereal disease declined overall, these infected men ensured that small and deadly pockets of disease remained a powerful threat.

Generally speaking, however, public health experts were justified in patting themselves on the back for their recent successes. The introduction of sulfa drugs and penicillin had led to steep declines in rates of both gonorrhea and syphilis, and it appeared that the battle against venereal disease could finally be won.

But if more effective treatments were at the heart of this decline in venereal disease, what role had education played?

At a basic level, the government's campaign had been instrumental in educating Americans about the dangers of venereal disease. This greater awareness had resulted not merely in "folks a-flockin'" to be tested for syphilis but in a willingness to devote substantial financial resources and efforts to the problem.[51] These resources had led, in turn, to major breakthroughs in the treatment of venereal disease. Having learned about and come to understand not only the problems that venereal disease caused but also how easily it could be cured, Americans were now willing to be tested and treated for these diseases.

The future looked bright.

CHAPTER FIVE

A FALSE SENSE OF SECURITY
1946-1959

Almost every case of syphilis, if brought under medical care
early enough, can be treated with penicillin quickly, easily, and
conveniently in a doctor's office or in a clinic.

CAUSE, SPREAD, AND CURE OF SYPHILIS, 1954

There is evidence that it is important to keep information
[about venereal disease] constantly before the public, to
maintain a sufficiently high level of knowledge.

EARLY SYPHILIS CASEFINDING THROUGH EDUCATION, 1950

I f you want to know the truth," seventeen-year-old Holden Caulfield confessed, "I'm a virgin." He had come "quite close to doing it a couple of
times," but as he reluctantly admitted, "something always happen[ed]" to
prevent it. "The thing is, most of the time you're coming close to doing it with
a girl—a girl that isn't a prostitute, I mean—she keeps telling you to stop . . .
[and] the trouble with me is, I stop," Holden lamented.[1] Outside the fictional
world of *The Catcher in the Rye*, Gwen Barnes, a young teenager in upstate New
York, struggled with problems that echoed those of J. D. Salinger's infamous an-
tihero. Throughout the 1950s Barnes and her steady boyfriend "had terrible
fights in the car . . . he'd push, push, push, push, I'd say stop, stop, stop—we
both knew the rules." Worried because "what I was doing was so bad and I was
enjoying it so much," Barnes fought to control her own sexual desires as well as
those of her boyfriend.[2]

Barnes showed unusual fortitude in resisting the urge to engage in sex. Many
of her peers did not. By 1957, teens' failure to "stop, stop, stop" had sent rates
of teenage pregnancies to record levels, unsurpassed even today. The impact of
this high level of teen sexual activity was not, however, always apparent to the
casual observer. Census reporting, which failed to count illegitimate pregnancies among teens who still lived with their parents, hid the reality of teen preg-

nancy from public view, as did the social convention that encouraged many eighteen- and nineteen-year-olds to marry when pregnant or simply when they decided to become sexually active. Adding to the problem was the social pressure that led many unmarried pregnant women to hide, or at least fail to acknowledge publicly, their pregnancies, especially if the child was being given up for adoption. The illegality and underground nature of abortion complicated the issue even further. Public health experts found it impossible to determine exactly how many abortions were performed each year. Estimates ranged between 200,000 and 1.2 million.[3] Because state laws overwhelmingly required couples to submit to blood tests before marrying, venereal disease was less easy to hide. In 1956, evidence from these tests, as well as more general epidemiological studies, revealed that rates of venereal disease, which had been declining among the general population, had now begun to climb among teenagers. Yet even as these worrisome trends were becoming evident, *Time* was heralding Americans' growing sophistication in using birth control to limit the size of their families and prevent unwanted pregnancies.[4]

Neither this growing acceptance of birth control nor the skyrocketing rates of teenage pregnancy and venereal disease translated into calls for better or even more sex education during the 1950s. The resulting scarcity of sex education programs has led some historians to argue that sex education was "virtually moribund" during this period.[5] But the federal government actually implemented aggressive and innovative techniques to control venereal disease throughout the 1950s, and education was a central component of these efforts. Federal officials also began to lay the foundations for what would become, in the 1960s and 1970s, an impressive family-planning program. Although the government and many of its private partners began to connect ongoing and new federally funded initiatives to expand sex education with the very real problem of teenage pregnancy during the 1940s and 1950s, the government's long history of using sex education to battle venereal disease meant that efforts to link sex education and preventing teenage pregnancy were often deemphasized or ignored during this period. By the early 1950s this disregard for sex education had become so extensive that Public Health Service officers were cautioning their fellow citizens against a "sense of false security." By 1957 this "sense of false security" had swelled to such a degree that serious and damaging cuts in the government's sex education program were being proposed and implemented.[6]

Going to the Chapel, Gonna Get Married

In 1957 a concerned reader wrote to the advice columnist Mary Haworth about a young woman who was about to give birth to an illegitimate child. The young woman's elderly relatives believed that "anyone who presumes to criticize her has committed a crime." Horrified by the family's lax attitude, the reader asked, "What chance does [this girl] have of becoming a well-adjusted citizen in view of the attitude her relatives have taken?" For Haworth, the answer was clear: "Careful consideration should be given to placing [the girl] in more favorable surroundings (if possible) in the future—to afford a more constructive, remedial 'social conditioning.'" It might also be beneficial, Haworth suggested, if the girl was forced to acknowledge her mistakes publicly. Haworth nevertheless admitted that the moral standards that would have led this girl to a public acknowledgment of her shame "aren't exactly in fashion today."[7]

In 1943, fourteen years before Haworth bemoaned America's declining moral values, the *Dallas Morning News* had bluntly warned that "many boys and girls will be cast adrift when peace comes."[8] The Dallas paper was not alone in making this prediction. During the decade and a half following V-J Day, fluctuating attitudes toward sex, birth control, marital relationships, and the family led to escalating concerns about Americans' sexual behavior and the strength of the American family. The release of Alfred Kinsey's groundbreaking studies *Sexual Behavior in the Human Male* (1947) and *Sexual Behavior in the Human Female* (1953) upped the ante by providing graphic evidence that Americans' sexual behavior did not reflect the principles most people endorsed. The overwhelming majority of American adult women, some 95 percent, had engaged in "petting" before marriage. Most shocking of all, 50 percent of American women had had premarital intercourse, and the vast majority of them were unrepentant about their decision to do so.

Concerned that "appeals to moral rectitude . . . were not likely to eradicate" early forms of sexual experimentation, public health professionals, social workers, and others began advocating that Americans marry early.[9] Federal initiatives, such as the GI Bill and relaxed mortgage lending practices, added an additional push by ensuring that Americans who wanted to marry young could afford to do so. Celebrating this trend toward early marriage as a positive development, editors of women's magazines such as *Women's Home Companion* now argued that "when two people are ready for sexual intercourse they are ready for marriage—and they *should* marry." Suddenly, not marrying had become "social cowardice," while Americans who questioned the wisdom of early marriages were told that "society has no right to stand in [the couple's] way."[10]

Beginning in the 1940s, young Americans responded to this social pressure by embarking on a nationwide rush to the altar. By 1951, Americans' average age at marriage had dropped significantly, with men marrying at the age of twenty-two and women at the age of twenty. These numbers remained low over the next decade; by 1959, almost half of all brides were under nineteen. While these changes reflected a broader trend toward marrying earlier that had begun some sixty years earlier, the drop in marital age that occurred in the 1950s was especially dramatic when compared with marital patterns just twenty years earlier. During the Depression, poverty-stricken Americans had married at a significantly older age than their counterparts would do in the postwar period.

This postwar trend toward early marriage shaped sex education programs. Throughout the late 1940s and 1950s, most sex education classes, whether taught in a high school or a college, focused on the role of sex *within* marriage. In some ways there was nothing new in this approach. The government's sex education programs had always advocated that Americans have sex within the confines of marriage, but now privately and publicly funded sex education began to prioritize a range of issues relating to the family. The "family life education" that emerged during this period provided lessons on such domestic tasks as managing a household budget. Lessons of this sort superseded or in some instances even replaced lessons on preventing venereal disease or illegitimate pregnancies.[11]

Families meant children, and throughout the postwar period Americans came to believe that parenthood should quickly follow marriage.[12] Whereas previous birth cohorts had married and had children at varied ages, American men and women who were born in the 1930s overwhelmingly began and completed their families before they were out of their twenties. The ensuing population explosion was less a consequence of families having more children than of couples all having their families at the same time. The result was that "the smallest birth cohort of twentieth-century women, those born in the 1930s, had the largest birth cohort of children: the baby boom."[13] Between 1946 and 1964, 76 million babies were born, with 4 million new babies "plopping out onto the changing mat every year." By the mid 1950s "there were," as one baby boomer has quipped, "always six hundred kids everywhere except where two or more neighborhoods met—at The Park, for instance—where the numbers would grow into the thousands."[14]

The Population Bomb

Ironically, the baby boom, which began in 1946 and continued unchecked until 1964, emerged in an era of growing sophistication regarding birth control. By the 1950s the modern birth control movement had a long history. Margaret Sanger had opened the first birth control clinic in Brooklyn in 1916. The clinic had operated illegally, as the Comstock Act forbade physicians and nurses from dispensing contraceptives or contraceptive advice. In 1936 a slight modification in the law opened the door for physicians to dispense not only information about contraceptives but contraceptives themselves. Although some thirty states retained on their books laws that made it illegal for physicians to provide contraceptive advice, residents in many areas of the country now had access to contraception.

On the surface, the lopsided nature of the baby boom, which had resulted in some 76 million babies being born during an eighteen-year period, might have made it appear that contraception was irrelevant to many women. But the structure of the boom actually led to increased calls for safe and effective birth control. Because American women overwhelmingly married and completed their families early, most women now faced fifteen or more years of fertility after they had decided to bear no more children. The widespread belief that a woman's happiness should be derived from her marriage and her family made many women reluctant to demand better access to safe and effective contraceptives during this period. However, ineffective contraception, which often resulted in unwanted pregnancies, meant that many married women were deeply unhappy with their birth control options. While this unhappiness was not always made public, married women, who possessed a moral authority that their unmarried counterparts lacked, were increasingly receptive to the idea of better and more effective birth control.[15]

During the postwar era, many married couples used condoms as their primary method of birth control. Condoms, which the Public Health Service had gingerly advocated as a means of preventing venereal disease in the 1930s, were sold over the counter. This allowed couples to buy them anonymously and without a prescription from a physician. Spermicidal jellies and douches had a similar appeal. Diaphragms, however, required that a woman be fitted by a physician. The American Medical Association had cautiously sanctioned physicians' providing contraceptive advice to married women, but women as well as physicians were often reluctant to discuss the subject. As a result, married women often shied away from using diaphragms. If the subject remained a difficult one for married women, it was an impossible one for unmarried women to discuss with their physicians.

During the 1920s and 1930s, the emergence of the birth control movement had both paralleled and reflected the emergence of eugenics. Not all eugenicists promoted birth control. In fact, many knew that the two groups they believed should be reproducing—the educated and the wealthy—were more likely to use birth control than the poor and the uneducated. But some eugenicists saw birth control as a means of controlling the fertility of the "deviant" or less desirable strains of American society. During the late 1940s, as the American eugenics movement foundered in the wake of the Holocaust and the forced sterilization policies of the Nazis, eugenicists began to lessen their emphasis on preventing the "unfit" from reproducing. Instead, they began to speak about ensuring the "quality of life" for all Americans. This assessment echoed the views of two other groups: general advocates of birth control, who saw choice as a means of ensuring that unwanted children no longer placed undue emotional and financial pressure on families, as well as advocates of population control. During the late 1940s and 1950s these three groups merged to become "the dominant voice for federal involvement in family planning policy in the early 1950s."[16]

Concerns about inequality and poverty led many proponents of population control to see family planning as the solution to America's, and the world's, social problems. In poorer regions of the United States, such as the rural South, early proponents of population control saw a strong link between poverty and large families of unwanted children. White Southerners who associated poverty with African Americans often accepted and endorsed efforts at population control, which they saw as fundamental to encouraging a decrease in the African-American population. There was one small catch, however. Contemporary public health experts noted that although white Southerners expressed enthusiasm for the use of birth control by African Americans, these whites were still more likely than their Northern counterparts to see "birth control [as] taboo as a subject for public or polite conversation."[17]

Frustrated by this stonewalling, proponents of population control looked to Puerto Rico for a better testing ground for federally funded initiatives to promote birth control. Federal officials had long seen the widespread poverty on the island as evidence that Puerto Rico was overpopulated. Although this assessment of the island's problems was shaped by imperialist and racist sentiments, these were not the only factors influencing federal attempts to promote family planning there. Early on, a committee on Puerto Rico had noted that "endeavors to improve the health conditions of Puerto Rico must be organically tied to and contingent upon effective birth control work."[18] Improving and alleviating poverty in Puerto Rico would, in other words, require that the federal government actively encourage the use of birth control. While this belief that birth control was central to alleviating poverty was focused first on Puerto Rico, the advent of the Depression led many public health and population control experts to view birth control as a means of addressing economic disparities across the country; the smaller the population, the easier it would be to ensure that workers received not only competitive wages but wages that could also allow them to feed, educate, and care for their children. In 1937, legislation to legalize birth control was introduced into Puerto Rico, and in 1942 the Public Health Service began to promote educational programs that encouraged the use of contraceptives in the territory.

On the surface, the rationale for these programs was to allow women to space their children in such a way as to enable them to support and educate the children they chose to have. But Puerto Rico's status as a territory, as opposed to a state, also meant that the federal government played a disproportionately large role in the governance of the island. Puerto Rico was the perfect testing ground for an innovative federal policy which promoted family planning by linking it to health care and the stability of the family unit. With its predominantly Catholic population, Puerto Rico also provided insight into the difficulties federally funded programs that promoted birth control could expect to encounter from religious groups. The success of these initiatives in Puerto Rico led many federal officials to begin advocating that similar initiatives be adopted on the mainland.

But despite the success of these measures, population control experts remained worried that faulty or ineffective contraceptive methods could undermine their efforts to educate families both on how to space their children and on how to have fewer children overall. During the 1950s the Population Council, a private foundation, fostered research into new contraceptives. Similarly, Planned Parenthood, a private organization founded in 1942, also funded research into a new oral contraceptive. By the mid-1950s Planned Parenthood had "stitched together the birth control movement and the population control movement into a virtually seamless fabric," and Americans overwhelmingly used "the terms 'birth control,' 'family planning' and 'population control' interchangeably."[19] In pursuit of these goals, Planned Parenthood helped to fund work by Gregory Goodwin Pincus, a biologist at the Worcester Foundation for

Experimental Biology in Massachusetts. Additional funding for this work was provided by Katherine McCormack, a wealthy widow whose husband had succumbed to schizophrenia a few years after their marriage. Although Pincus' work was directly related to what was emerging as a focus on family planning by the federal government, neither the National Science Foundation nor the National Institutes of Health funded Pincus' work during the 1950s.

Because Massachusetts law forbade the use of contraceptives, the pill that Pincus developed in 1956 was tested in Puerto Rico. Like federal officials who had viewed Puerto Rico as the perfect testing ground for federally funded initiatives promoting family planning, Pincus saw the island as providing the perfect site for testing his oral contraceptive. As an overpopulated "prototype underdeveloped country on America's own doorstep," Puerto Rico was widely viewed as needing effective family planning methods more than any other region of the United States.[20] Additionally, because Puerto Rican women tended to possess lower levels of education than their mainland counterparts, testing the pill there would provide insights into whether use of the pill would require extensive training or education. Finally, testing the drug in Puerto Rico had the added benefit of allowing Pincus to avoid extensive press scrutiny from the country's more prominent newspapers, all of which were located stateside. Field tests for the drug were not without controversy, but by 1959, results indicated that Pincus' oral contraceptive was safe, effective, and very easy to use. In May of 1960 the Food and Drug Administration (FDA) formally approved the birth control pill, paving the way for the federal government to promote comprehensive family planning initiatives, which advocated the use of safe and easy-to-use contraceptives.

But in 1950, all this was still in the future. Throughout the 1950s, as the federal government tentatively began to raise the idea of family planning and to link this idea to the broader goal of ending poverty, most Americans remained unaware of the sharp turn that federally funded sex education programs had taken. It would not be until the 1960s that federally funded educational initiatives promoting family planning would reach all Americans.

"Sly, Lewd—in Plain Fact, Dirty"

During the postwar period Americans' emphasis on family and domesticity was accompanied by growing concerns about morality. Reflecting these concerns, Americans became increasingly willing to identify with a specific religion. This embrace of religion did not mean that "degeneracy" or worries about degeneracy declined. Moralists, many of them linked to the Catholic Church or to different Protestant sects, found evidence of depravity everywhere. Hollywood provided, as it always had, especially graphic evidence of degeneracy, and throughout the 1950s significant numbers of religious leaders lectured their congregants on the dangers of Hollywood's sexually explicit films. In 1956 these concerns exploded over the release of *Baby Doll*, a film written by the award-winning playwright Tennessee Williams. A reviewer for *Time* described the film as "possibly the dirtiest American-made motion picture that has ever been legally exhibited." The film opened to bomb threats and threats of mass boycotts in small cities such as Hartford and Albany. In that hotbed of vice, New York City, Cardinal Francis Spellman found himself "exhort[ing] Catholic people from patronizing this film under pain of sin." All this commotion led, of course, to walloping ticket sales, which *Variety* characterized as "Huge, Sock, Whopping and Terrif."[21]

The furor over *Baby Doll* was not unique. Throughout the postwar period the Legion of Decency condemned many films as "vile and unwholesome" and asked Catholics to take an oath to boycott films that the Legion condemned as "a grave menace to youth, to home life, to country and religion."[22] Few Americans were prepared to buck these calls for public denunciations. In her highly autobiographical novel about growing up in the 1950s, Caryl Rivers describes her teenage heroine's decision to ignore the Legion's call to boycott Jane Russell films as one not made lightly. Rivers' character notes dryly that Jane Russell's breasts "certainly weren't a Near Occasion of Sin for me; they left me cold," and she says that her desire to be a journalist led her to disagree with the Legion's calls for censorship. Yet nonconformity proves to be extraordinarily difficult. Rivers' character sums up the import of her actions in these words: "I have done a few brave things in my life since then—I have been where guns were fired uncomfortably near me in anger and I did my job . . . but I never did anything as hard as not getting to my feet in Church to recite the Legion of Decency pledge when I was a senior at Immaculate Heart High School."[23]

Actions that were viewed as nonconforming usually existed within tightly confined and controlled circumstances. Characterized by Frank Sinatra as having "imbecile reiterations and sly, lewd—in plain fact, dirty—lyrics," rock 'n' roll was perhaps the best example of this type of nonconformist conformity. Rock 'n' roll brought fears of a generation actively rebelling against its elders, but it was also a multimillion-dollar industry.[24] Elvis Presley's wildly swinging hips notwithstanding, most rock of the 1950s was fairly tame, especially in its references to sex, but the concerns it evoked reflected a broader fear of teenagers themselves. Films such as *The Wild Ones, West Side Story, Blackboard Jungle,* and *Rebel without a Cause* all hinted that teenagers, a term that had only recently been coined, were living lives that defied social norms. News stories about teenagers petting in parked cars abounded, as did stories about violent juvenile delinquents. Given the fact that rates of juvenile delinquency remained low throughout this period, these stories about youth violence did not reflect the reality of postwar society. However, stories about teenagers engaging in sex often did have the ring of truth. Teenagers, as Gwen Barnes and Holden Caulfield could attest, did indeed engage in sex, but large numbers of them married either when they began to engage in sex or shortly after initiating sex. In a sharp contrast to today, when the practice of teenage marriage raises serious concerns, postwar Americans expressed no real concerns regarding the relative youth of those who married and embarked on parenthood. In fact, once teens married and had children, worries about their behavior completely ceased. As the editor of *Better Homes and Gardens* happily put it, when "there are three in [a] family," there is no need to worry about a couple.[25]

Above and beyond the threats posed by unmarried teens, rock 'n' roll, and the film industry, there were very real reasons for fear in the 1950s. The emergence of the Cold War, following first the detonation of the atom bomb in 1945 and then the hydrogen bomb in 1952, sparked concerns that a new world war was imminent. The upsurge in patriotism that emerged as a result of both the nuclear arms race and the ill-defined threat of communism provided little relief. Stoked by the fear-mongering tactics of Senator Joe McCarthy, this intense patriotism translated into a reluctance to acknowledge or look critically at the problems that plagued postwar America. And there were problems.

Jim Crow laws sharply limited the lives of African Americans across the South, causing poverty and misery. In the North the situation was little better; widespread prejudices and limited opportunities trapped many African Americans in the nation's urban slums. Among the many rationales that Americans developed to justify their prejudices was an age-old belief that African Americans were sexually promiscuous. In the 1950s, as the civil rights movement began to challenge Jim Crow, white Americans' fears about the sexual threat posed by African Americans and other nonwhites exploded. This was the decade in which Emmett Till was infamously tortured and killed for allegedly whistling at a white woman in Mississippi. Other less well-known incidents also inflamed these fears. In 1948, for example, the local paper in Anniston, Alabama, high-lighted a story out of Milwaukee about "widespread sex orgies between white girls, Negro youths and perverts." Lest white readers of this article believe that African Americans were unique in lusting after white girls, the accompanying article discussed a white slavery ring in Shanghai.[26]

Adding to Americans' worries about sex were a growing number of articles discussing homosexuality, its causes, and its prevalence. Poorly understood at the time, homosexuality was defined as a form of mental illness, and acts associated with homosexuality were illegal in many states. The upheavals of the war had, however, led to the "genesis of a gay awakening . . . [as] gay people found opportunities to meet each other" in both sex-segregated military units and factories.[27] While most homosexuals and lesbians remained deeply closeted during this period, homosexuality was more evident than at previous times in American history. To postwar Americans who were unaccustomed either to candid discussions about sexual orientation or to evidence of nonheterosexual behavior, homosexuality appeared to be everywhere. Overwhelmed by what they incorrectly perceived as a dramatic rise in homosexuality, many Americans now saw this type of sexual behavior as a direct threat to their own families and the nation at large.

Moralists' outrage over what they viewed as sexually explicit films or music meant that Americans were often forced to acknowledge the complex role sex played in their society. But the focus on vague threats such as those posed by Hollywood and the music industry often deflected Americans from looking deeply at venereal disease and teenage pregnancy, both of which were becoming real problems during this period. The reluctance to acknowledge these problems meant, in turn, that Americans were unprepared to fund and support federal initiatives to promote sex education throughout this period, even as the problems associated with Americans' sexual behavior became increasingly evident to public health experts.

Detectives on the Case

As the war wound down, "DDT, the wonder insecticide, which has been second only to penicillin," became "the biggest continuing science news [story] of 1944." The widespread use of DDT, which killed the mosquitos that carried malaria, eradicated malaria in the United States—no small feat in a nation that had always been plagued by the disease.[28] Only two years before the mainstream

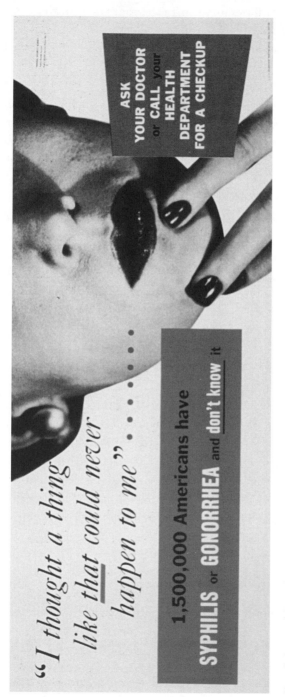

Even "nice people" caught and spread venereal disease (1952). Department of Health and Human Services.

media heralded the introduction of DDT, the Public Health Service had launched a program to protect Americans, specifically soldiers, from the disease. Given the awkward name of Malaria Control in War Areas (MCWA), this new PHS program was headquartered away from Washington, in the heart of malaria country. Working from a base in Atlanta, PHS officers focused on controlling malaria in fifteen Southern states, Puerto Rico, and the Virgin Islands. Initially work on this project was slow, but in 1943, mass spraying with DDT radically limited and arrested the spread of malaria. In the ordinary course of events, the retreat of malaria would have led to the successful and permanent termination of MCWA, but Surgeon General Thomas Parran believed that MCWA could fill a broader role than simply tracking and eradicating malaria.

Parran had the authority to expand and transform MCWA, but any transformation of the program would require the continuation of federal funding. In 1946 the Public Health Service received sufficient funding to enable MCWA to expand its original mission. The MCWA also received a new name, the Communicable Disease Center (CDC). Headquartered in Atlanta, the CDC was specifically tasked with tracking and controlling communicable diseases, an assignment that included tracking venereal disease.

Raymond Vonderlehr, the director of the Venereal Disease Division under Parran, was appointed as one of the first directors of the new CDC. Vonderlehr had worked closely with Surgeon General Parran, whom he also considered a close friend. Like Parran, Vonderhelr had been publicly critical of the military's campaign to control venereal disease. But unlike Parran, Vonderlehr had suffered professionally as a result; he had been exiled to Puerto Rico where he supervised one of the Public Health Service's ten regions. In 1947 the opportunity to head a new agency, one whose overall mission reflected his own interests in venereal disease, led Vonderlehr to accept the directorship. With this appointment it looked as though venereal disease control would become a high priority with the CDC. But despite Vonderlehr's background in fighting venereal disease and despite the fact that CDC's second director, Theodore Bauer, also came out of the Venereal Disease Division, venereal disease did not become a central priority with this new agency in the 1950s.

The Venereal Disease Division was, however, formally transferred to the CDC during this period. One of its directors enthused that this division's workers were "the most dedicated group of all [in CDC]—competent *and* dedicated."[29] But it was not just enthusiasm that shaped the actions taken by the Venereal Disease Division. Innovative approaches to public health were also central in transforming the division and its efforts to limit the spread of venereal disease. In 1948 Lida J. Usilton, who had been working on sex education programs in the Public Health Service since the 1920s, drew on the ideas of Alfred Kinsey to create an innovative program to track the spread of venereal disease and the prevalence of risky sexual behavior. Kinsey's researchers had conducted extensive interviews to track patterns of sexual activity. They then compiled lists of their interviewees' sexual partners and interviewed all of them, creating an interconnected web of sexual contacts. Adopting Kinsey's methods, the CDC trained young college graduates to interview patients suffering from venereal disease, to track down their sexual contacts, and to persuade those suffering from venereal disease, along with their sexual contacts, to undergo treatment. These new disease detectives were called Public Health Advisors (PHAs). Previously federally funded educational programs had been aimed at a broad audience, but the introduction of PHAs radically transformed these initiatives. Now the CDC could specifically direct educational programs at those who were suffering from venereal disease or at risk of contracting syphilis or gonorrhea. Within a few years the new program had become extraordinarily successful at lowering the incidence of venereal disease. In fact, its success was such that "in 1953, the Eisenhower administration proposed the elimination of the venereal disease program on the grounds that the job had been done."[30]

For congressional legislators and federal budget directors, the proposed elimination of funding for the venereal disease program made sense: why fund education if other methods were more effective at controlling venereal disease? But the CDC and the Public Health Service held firm. When patients were asked what was "most helpful in getting people to" undergo testing for syphilis, significant percentages of people said education—proof, the PHS believed, that educational programs should still be viewed as the lynchpin of any venereal disease program.[31] Although the Public Health Service managed to mount an extensive defense for the program, funding for education—and the battle against venereal disease—radically declined during this period. This decline did not, however, result in a termination of the CDC's efforts to eradicate venereal disease; the Public Health Service's insistence that the battle had not yet been won provided the program with a limited reprieve. However, the cuts that were enacted were deep enough to limit the war against venereal disease. Much to the horror of public health experts, venereal disease rates began rising shortly after the budget cuts were enacted. Rates of teenage pregnancy, which the PHS still failed to see as a real problem, also remained extremely high during this period.

There were some bright spots. The creation of the CDC pushed the federal government to track and assess, routinely and accurately, rates of both venereal disease and teenage pregnancy. More important, it also forced the government to consider these problems within the broader context of communicable diseases and public health, something Surgeon General Thomas Parran had long advocated.

Outside of Atlanta other federal agencies were also changing the practice of public health. In 1944 the passage of the Public Health Service Act had expanded the Commissioned Corps of the Public Health Service, with the result that the Corps grew from 625 officers in 1940 to 2,600 in 1945. The number of civilians working for the PHS also grew to 16,000 in this same period.[32] This was no bloated federal bureaucracy; the growth in staff was accompanied by an expansion of the mission and tasks the PHS directed. As global health became increasingly important, the PHS began to track diseases such as syphilis and gonorrhea as they moved across the world. Along with the development of large-scale epidemiological studies, the government also radically increased its commitment to research the causes, nature, and treatment of diseases. Throughout the war the research arm of the Public Health Service, the National Institutes of Health, had received enormous budgets. Even before the war had begun, NIH had moved to a large campus in Bethesda, Maryland; this new campus provided space for the agency to grow, and by the late 1940s the NIH campus was the site of some of the most ground-breaking biomedical research in the United States. The program's success, as well as its willingness to hire female scientists as well as married couples, meant that the agency also became a haven for some of the nation's most accomplished scientists.[33] To pay for this research, NIH's budget grew at astronomical rates during the postwar period, swelling from a low of $8 million in 1947 to $1 billion in 1966. These budget increases enabled NIH scientists, or scientists funded by NIH grants, to launch a variety of long-term and highly complex research projects.[34] Understanding of the causes and consequences of venereal diseases and illegitimate pregnancies benefited directly from this upsurge in funding, but this increase also had consequences for the long term as well. Some forty years after NIH became the nation's premier biomedical research institution, its scientists would lead research into a new sexually transmitted disease, AIDS.

In 1955 the Public Health Service expanded yet again when it absorbed another federal agency, the Indian Health Service (IHS). PHS physicians had always provided merchant marines with medical care, but the inclusion of the IHS within the PHS brought still more Public Health Service physicians into contact with patients on a daily basis. This work expanded some PHS officers' understanding of how and why patients responded to different educational programs and treatment. More important, working in some of the nation's poorest and most segregated communities led PHS physicians to think broadly about the health needs of minority communities as well as the connections between poverty and "social" problems such as venereal disease and illegitimacy. Obviously, the continuation of the notorious Tuskegee Syphilis Experiment during this period graphically demonstrates that this new work did not directly or immediately translate into greater sensitivity on the part of federal officials. Nonetheless, the incorporation of the IHS within the Public Health Service ultimately led to a more sophisticated understanding of the role that cultural sensitivity played in disease remediation. In the 1960s and 1970s this emphasis on greater cultural sensitivity would lead to better and more targeted educational campaigns.

In the short term, however, the Public Health Service failed to address the public health needs of the nation's minority communities. The most spectacular of these failures was in the African-American community. Since 1921 the PHS had worked as a partner in the National Negro Health Movement, a program spearheaded by Booker T. Washington and intended to improve African Americans' health. Despite this partnership, the federal government's track record in promoting and improving public health among African-American communities continued to be poor. In the program's early years, no less a PHS luminary than Raymond Vonderlehr had maintained that "quite obviously the color line cannot be drawn where the prevention of disease is concerned." Yet the federal government's public health activities reflected the prejudices of the broader American society. These prejudices had led, most infamously, to the Tuskegee Syphilis Experiment, but they also caused lesser known setbacks for minority health. In 1951 the premature death of the National Negro Health Movement ensured that the PHS abandoned even its lukewarm commitment to address the health concerns of the African-American community. While the reasons for the program's termination were varied and reflected changing perceptions of segregation, the program's early demise prevented the Public Health Service from taking a critical and unprejudiced look at the public health problems caused by poverty, Jim Crow, and the nation's centuries-old legacy of prejudice toward African Americans.[35]

When the National Negro Health Movement collapsed, the Public Health Service was nurturing new programs in its new agencies. The addition of these new programs did not immediately result in the radical transformation of federally funded sex education campaigns, but they did lay the groundwork for a better and more comprehensive understanding of venereal disease and teenage pregnancy in the decades that followed. And this better understanding would prove crucial in the battle against sexual ignorance during the 1960s and 1970s.

Father Doesn't Know Best

Four years after the end of the war, Fritz Redi, a member of the Public Health Service's Commission on Mental Health, soberly noted that "sex crimes and the attitudes of the nation's youth" are "the fault of the parents." Pointing out that "parents, church leaders, and counselors ward off questions concerning sex," Redi lectured public health experts and educators in Cleveland, saying that sex education should "begin when a child starts asking questions."[36] Just a year before Redi's speech, a widely publicized report had indicated that children's "greatest sources of sex information come from friends of their own age and older boys and girls."[37] There was nothing new in either the report or the lecture; since 1918 the Public Health Service had complained that parents' failure to provide sex education caused their children to turn to "disreputable" sources, and the biased information children received from these sources fostered unhealthy attitudes toward sex.

Although the practice of venereal disease control had shifted with the introduction of penicillin and more aggressive epidemiological techniques, the federal government's sex education programs continued to be mired in the concerns and practices of the prewar era. Eager to put to rest the belief that penicillin had eradicated not only venereal disease but also the need for sex education, the Public Health Service announced that it would be launching a new sex education campaign in 1950. But rather than emphasizing concerns about high rates of teenage and illegitimate pregnancy or pointing out that good sex education was simply a part of good public health education, the government pitched this new sex education campaign as yet another battle to combat venereal disease. Americans responded with apathy. Even the sobering statistic of 100,000 children still being born each year with congenital syphilis failed to energize people for this "new" campaign. Well aware of the wonders of penicillin,

Americans simply did not see venereal disease as an urgent concern, and because venereal disease was still promoted as the primary reason for promoting sex education, sex education seemed irrelevant.

The campaign "launched" in 1950 was simply a continuation of the ongoing program of educational outreach that had been initiated during and immediately after the war. In 1949, for example, a year before its "new" sex education campaign was heralded in the media, the Public Health Service had implemented an intensive educational program in Philadelphia. Directed at specific neighborhoods where the incidence and prevalence of venereal disease were believed to be especially high, the campaign used "spectacular displays" to grab the attention of Philadelphians. Blimps with illuminated messages, street banners, and even trucks with loudspeakers broadcasting information about venereal disease were seen and heard by thousands of the city's residents.[38] In smaller towns and cities where the use of a blimp or illuminated messages was not cost-effective, public education programs continued to be a dreary repetition of programs used throughout the 1920s and 1930s. In 1949, for example, residents in Annapolis, Maryland, found themselves sitting once again in the local Elks Lodge as "educators, clergymen, doctors, dentists, pharmacists, and other community figures" lectured them on the dangers of venereal disease. The only remotely interesting moment came when a representative of the Public Health Service showed both *Know for Sure*, the sexually graphic film on venereal disease that had become a standard tool in the government's arsenal against sexual ignorance, and *Human Growth*, a film about sex intended for adolescents. The discussion that followed did little to nothing in terms of sparking community action or even encouraging parents and local community leaders to provide comprehensive sex education in the home, church, or community center.[39]

Blimps aside, the government had little new to offer. By the 1950s, "lectures, films, filmstrips, pamphlets, comic booklets, posters, and portable exhibits" had all been used to promote sex education for decades. Even the use of television, the most innovative aspect of these new campaigns, was not really new. Its use was more a reflection of the government's age-old belief that all "channels of communication . . . [should be] used to get the information to the public" than a daringly new method of educating Americans.[40] Moreover, federal officials might pride themselves on the importance of exploiting all "channels of communication," but even they knew that such methods had their limitations. Educational spots did, it was true, encourage Americans to be tested for venereal disease, but these sex education messages needed to be constantly updated and reiterated if they were to be effective. Constantly updating and playing these messages cost money, which the Public Health Service did not possess.

Just as there was nothing new in how the government pitched sex education, so too was there nothing new in the message being promoted. During the postwar era the government continued to rely heavily on materials produced before or during the war. One of the more widely circulated pamphlets during this period was *The Causes, Spread, and Cure of Syphilis.* This pamphlet differed from similarly named pamphlets that had been produced before the war only in its discussion of penicillin. The films that were shown in Annapolis and elsewhere were similarly dated, and the messages the PHS promoted on the radio and on television had been for the most part formulated during the war.

Concerned that Americans were dismissing the federal government's sex education program as the "same old same old," some communities attempted to generate interest in the subject by linking the need for sex education to broader concerns in American society. In Chester, Pennsylvania, for example, community leaders pitched sex education as a patriotic duty and a means of fighting communism. Proclaiming that the "family unit . . . bulwarked by proper, moral, ethical and sex education . . . [is] the most effective protection for America against foreign ideologies which are the opposite of this country's principle of democracy," participants in community discussions argued that sex education was needed if America was to remain safe from the Red Menace.[41]

Sex education was pitched as not only patriotic but also "scientific." Although federally funded programs had often advocated extremely moralistic or "Victorian" views of sex, federal officials had always insisted that the government's sex education materials were "scientific." Those who opposed the distribution of these materials were routinely branded as opposed to science. In the postwar period, when Americans' confidence in science and technology were at all-time highs, this emphasis on science seemed to promise that the government's educational materials were up to date and modern—even when they were not. But given Americans' love of science during this period, this approach found support at the grass-roots level. Few Americans were willing to come down against science and against sex education when Walter Winchell, a well-known news commentator and a strong promoter of the Public Health Service's campaign for sex education, intoned, "Science knows the cause [of venereal disease]. Science knows the cure. But ignorance . . . stands in the path of progress."[42]

Poll after poll had demonstrated and, the Public Health Service knew, that the majority of Americans wanted sex education to be taught in their communities and in their schools. The real debate centered, more often than not, on the type of sex education Americans believed should be made available. Although federal officials did not openly discuss local opposition to comprehensive sex education in any great detail, they believed that this opposition often stemmed more from Americans' failure to be honest about their own behavior than from any deep opposition to the overall idea of sex education per se. In heavily Mormon Utah, denial ran deep. There the Ogden paper promoted sex education and sought to quash fears that the "short and comparatively easy treatment [provided by penicillin] will have an effect on promiscuity." But while public health experts encouraged Utahans to endorse sex education, they noted that the state's residents were so morally upright that the concerns sex education might raise in some communities were irrelevant in Utah; Utahans didn't really need comprehensive sex education, in other words.[43] Utahans were not unique in promoting themselves as the most upright of the nations' citizens. Nearly every community, including New York City, cast itself as more upright or more honest than its neighbors and as being at the forefront of disease control. Small wonder, then, that many of the nation's citizens found themselves reluctant to fund and aggressively promote sex education programs in their own communities; it was neighboring communities, not their own, that needed comprehensive sex education.

Adding to these problems were the contradictory messages regarding sex that were ubiquitous in the postwar period. In Holland, Michigan, for example, the local paper's article on Fritz Redi's call for better and more comprehensive sex education appeared alongside an article and photo delighting in the new and revealing bikini styles that the paper termed "stripe tease" wear.[44] In the face of such contradictions, the Public Health Service glumly acknowledged that education had its limits, especially when it came to motivating Americans into safer sexual behavior.[45]

A Breath of Fresh Air

In 1956 the Public Health Service released alarming news that shook the nation: teenagers now accounted for almost half of all new cases of syphilis and gonorrhea. "Promiscuity," Abraham Gelperin, a public health expert, noted with dismay, "is somehow accepted as a natural part of growing up." Ignorance and contempt for syphilis and gonorrhea among the nation's young simply added to this growing acceptance of promiscuity. By February 1956, state officials and the nation's leading venereal disease associations were calling for "a big federal aid program to maintain a nation-wide control program."[46]

But the federal government had long maintained exactly such a program. In fact, during the late 1950s, while Americans clucked over the rising rates of venereal disease and spoke wistfully of national programs, the Public Health Service's nationwide control program was entering its fourth decade. As part of this work the government had already embarked on a new and more comprehensive attempt to document and understand the causes of risky sexual behavior among teens. By 1960, federally funded research had uncovered some disturbing trends: women, for example, were more likely to contract venereal disease at eighteen years of age than at any other age. Teenage girls, in other words, were more prone to engage in risky sexual behavior than their adult counterparts. Equally troubling was the realization that the younger a man was when he became sexually active, the more likely he was to engage in risky sexual behavior, with multiple partners. But most disturbing of all was the discovery that

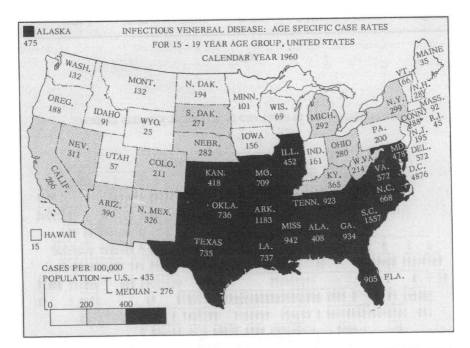

Federal agencies were beginning to uncover disturbing trends. *The Eradication of Syphilis: A Task Force Report to the Surgeon General Public Health Service on Syphilis Control in the United States* (1962). Department of Health and Human Services.

the problems associated with unprotected sex were "not confined to any sex, race, social group or section of the country."[47]

The government's investigations into the nature of Americans' sexual behavior reflected Alfred Kinsey's groundbreaking work, which had emphasized the importance of extensive and comprehensive interviews regarding patients' sexual histories. Kinsey's work, and to a lesser degree the government's findings, were forcing Americans to acknowledge that sex education was a very real necessity, given the realities of Americans' sexual behavior. In 1959 and 1960, as overall rates of venereal disease rose across the nation, the CDC called for a new war on sexual ignorance. Like previous campaigns for sex education, this new program would target all Americans. It would also include a directed sex education program aimed specifically at the nation's large population of adolescents. It would address not only venereal disease but also the issues of illegitimate and teenage pregnancy.

As the federal government began to look more closely at rising rates of venereal disease and illegitimate birth, a broader threat loomed. In 1951, Holden Caulfield, the anti-hero of J. D. Salinger's novel *The Catcher in the Rye*, ran away to New York City, where he encountered a world of vice and temptation in the form of prostitutes and sexually promiscuous women. At the time, Holden's adolescent rebellion was seen as an aberration. But by 1961 Holden had achieved iconic stature in American culture, and his sexual exploits, which had been viewed with such dismay ten years earlier, would come to be seen as minor when compared with those of his real-life counterparts, the baby boomers.

CHAPTER SIX

MAKING LOVE, NOT BABIES OR DISEASE 1960–1980

We have played a hypocritical game for years.
ROBERT FINCH, SECRETARY OF THE DEPARTMENT
OF HEALTH, EDUCATION, AND WELFARE, 1969

We can make sure that there is a place where sexually active
teenage boys and girls can receive reliable information.
TEENAGE PREGNANCY: EVERYONE'S PROBLEM, 1977

W hen the Beatles asked, "Why don't we do it in the road?" they promised that "no one will be watching us." But when John Lennon and
Yoko Ono posed naked on the cover of *Rolling Stone*, everyone was
watching. By 1969 sex had become, if not a public activity, then certainly a topic
of public discussion.

Only ten years before the Beatles teasingly suggested that sex could be public, American society had been quite different. From Maine to the new state of
Hawaii, Americans married early. In 1959 nearly half of all American women
were married by the age of nineteen, and half of those women became pregnant
within the first year of their marriage. Outwardly Americans deplored premarital sex and what they viewed as its two costly companions: disease and illegitimate births. But behind the drawn curtains of their homes, Americans often indulged in sex outside of marriage. By 1960 this covert sex had led to a rise in
illegitimacy rates and sexually transmitted diseases. It had also led to timid but
increasingly vocal calls for better access to birth control and more effective
methods for preventing conception.[1]

During the early part of the 1960s a series of widely publicized studies and
court cases led Americans to confront the discrepancy between their public
stance on sex and their actual behavior. This discrepancy was especially obvious

in Connecticut. There, married couples were legally forbidden to use contraceptives even within the privacy of their homes. Yet Connecticut boasted one of the lowest birth rates in the nation. In 1961, C. Lee Buxton, a physician frustrated by his inability to provide his patients with legal advice about contraception, initiated a court case challenging Connecticut's ban. The case, which was rapidly followed by other similar cases, pushed discussions of sex and contraception to the forefront of American public life.[2]

As Americans began to discuss contraceptives more openly, the Public Health Service rushed to assure teenagers that venereal diseases were also no longer "a 'hush-hush' subject" in American society.[3] While this statement reflected a great deal of wishful thinking, Americans' growing willingness to talk about sex and sexuality did translate to a growing readiness to discuss, or at least acknowledge, the problem of venereal disease. And venereal disease was indeed a growing problem. Beginning in 1957, rates of venereal disease had begun to rise at a threefold rate. For public health experts who had believed that penicillin would spell the death of syphilis and gonorrhea, the continued presence of these diseases was bad enough, but now the diseases were actually increasing at an alarming rate. Appalled by this state of affairs, the House Appropriations Committee testily demanded that the Public Health Service provide "recommendations for an effective program" to eradicate venereal disease.

In response to this demand, the Service fell back on the well-tested approach of all government agencies: it formed a task force. On September 31, 1961, the task force headed by Dr. Leona Baumgartner, New York City's commissioner of health, met for the first time to "recommend a course of action which would lead to the eradication of" venereal disease. If the actions taken by the government could also lead to a drop in illegitimacy rates, so much the better.

To the five members of the task force, the future looked bright. True, "no public health effort in modern times" had failed more completely than the battle to combat sexual ignorance. But reflecting the optimism that shaped the race to the moon as well as the battle to eradicate smallpox, the task force judged this new challenge to be "feasible."[4]

During the early 1960s, federal officials became convinced that ending poverty was also "feasible." Believing that unwanted and out-of-wedlock pregnancies caused and exacerbated poverty, public health experts pointed an accusatory finger at Americans' limited understanding and use of birth control. If Johnson's War on Poverty were to succeed, American women needed both to learn about birth control and to have access to safe and reliable contraception.

Growing concerns about population control as well as changing perceptions of sex and sexuality simply added to this push to educate Americans about birth control.[5]

The sex education materials that emerged in response to these new concerns were more frank than any of the Public Health Service's previous attempts at sex education. But for public health experts, the key question remained: Would these new campaigns be any more effective?

Are You Trying to Seduce Me, Mrs. Robinson?

When Linda LeClair opted to live with her boyfriend, she was a student at Barnard College. She was also part of a growing trend, one that fascinated newspaper readers and editors. In 1968 the *New York Times* published an article exploring this trend. Concerned that not all Americans approved of the actions of LeClair and her peers, the paper gave the interviewed couples pseudonyms. But within days of the story's appearance, an overheated public had ferreted out the identity of LeClair, and she found herself besieged by letters condemning her as a whore. Yet even as outraged Americans called for Barnard to expel her, LeClair and her fellow students were redefining American attitudes toward sex and sexuality.[6] By the late 1960s, conflicts such as the one LeClair had precipitated by admitting that she lived with her boyfriend had become so widespread that Americans had begun to speak of a sexual revolution.[7]

Judged in hindsight, the "revolution" that occurred during the 1960s and 1970s was nowhere near as rapid or radical as many Americans currently believe. In many ways the social changes that occurred during this period were the culmination of decades of quiet agitation by diverse groups across America. Additionally, the changes that *did* occur often had little to do with the highly publicized events that Americans today commonly associate with this period. Women did not burn their bras in public while demanding to be liberated.[8] "Key parties" in which partygoers engaged in sex with strangers did not suddenly invade the suburbs.[9] No doubt to the dismay of many students, Ronald Reagan's assertion that the Berkeley campus was dominated by orgies was untrue. And the double standard that judged men's and women's sexual behavior differently did not disappear.

Even the nation's foremost "revolutionaries" remained fairly conservative on sexual matters. Stokely Carmichael, the president of the radical Student Non-Violent Coordinating Committee, may have famously quipped that "the only position for women . . . is prone," but Carmichael's views simply reflected those of both the broader culture and many of his fellow radicals. Throughout the 1960s and 1970s the overwhelming majority of Americans, regardless of their political leanings, continued to regard marriage as the natural and preferred outcome for male-female relationships, and homophobia remained so ubiquitous that most liberal and radical Americans failed even to see it as an issue.

Although the 1960s and 1970s did not spark an unexpected and immediate "boom" in how Americans viewed sex and sexuality, the twenty years between 1959 and 1979 were characterized by significant changes. The death of curfews imposed on female college students, the growing availability of the pill for married *and* unmarried women, the legalization of abortion, an increasing recognition that women were not responsible for rape, the legalization of interracial marriage, and a rejection of the belief that homosexuality was a form of mental illness all transformed both how Americans behaved in private and how they viewed this behavior.

These concrete changes were also accompanied by a broader shift in American thinking on sex and sexuality that is more difficult to define. In the 1950s the vast majority of Americans condemned premarital sex—despite the fact that they often engaged in it. Twenty years later premarital sex was still widely viewed with anxiety and disapproval, but women who engaged in it were no longer shunned by neighbors or relatives. Similarly, unmarried couples could now freely check in to hotels and, more important, rent or buy property without any significant problems.[10]

Attitudes toward other types of sexual behavior also began shifting. In the 1950s, divorce, which did occur, was viewed as taboo and often discussed only in whispers. But by the 1970s, divorce was no longer social suicide for either women or men. As part of this broader trend, remarriages and blended families became more common. From *The Brady Bunch* to Judy Blume's *It's Not the End of the World*, blended and divorced families began to appear in popular culture. More surprising still, while television shows had always showed married couples sleeping in separate beds during the 1950s, television producers now acknowledged that adults had sex and allowed Carol and Mike Brady to share a bed.[11] Similarly, in 1960, when the birth control pill was approved by the Food and Drug Administration, many Americans, especially Catholics, were uneasy about the ethics of birth control. But by the 1970s the use of the pill was common among married and unmarried women, and its use was no longer viewed as a highly divisive issue. Even Pope Paul VI's encyclical *Humanae Vitae*, which condemned the use of birth control, did little to stop a growing number of Catholics from using it.[12]

At heart, then, the sexual revolution was less about Americans adopting radically new and strange ideas about sex than it was about Americans confronting the contradictions between their private behavior and their public responses to this behavior. For public health experts, the nation's growing willingness to discuss traditionally secret practices seemed to present a bonanza. Just as the sexual revolution of the late 1910s and 1920s had allowed the Public Health Service to speak more openly about venereal disease, so too did the sexual revolution of the 1960s and 1970s seem to presage an age in which Americans would awaken to and candidly discuss the public health implications of their sexual behavior.

A Time for Greatness?

Orgies. Riots. Marches. Tear gas. Most Americans remember the 1960s and 1970s as a time of incredible upheaval. But the period was more complex than these simple images imply. For many people the harsh reality of Vietnam, the use of chemical warfare in Southeast Asia, growing fears about nuclear war, Watergate, and the riots that shook the nation's inner cities and campuses translated into a growing distrust of their fellow citizens and government. Yet even as many Americans began to question their government and its intentions, this period also witnessed a growing belief that government experts could and should use science to eradicate poverty, disease, and even racial discrimination.

Federal officials shared this confidence, and the belief in the power of government and science was especially pervasive in the Department of Health, Education, and Welfare (HEW), the home of the Public Health Service. The decades preceding the 1960s had seen a substantial growth in the power and budgets of the PHS as its agencies, the CDC (Communicable Disease Center), the NIH (National Institutes of Health), and the FDA (Food and Drug Administration), expanded. Adding to this growing power was a dramatic surge in the number and quality of the personnel within the PHS itself.[13] The PHS had always attracted some of the nation's best physicians, but the Korean and Vietnam wars provided male physicians with an opportunity to complete their military service by serving in the Public Health Service as opposed to overseas. Many physicians entered the PHS to escape the draft, only to become so interested in the issue of public health that they elected to remain in the PHS long after their tours of duty expired. Conversely, those physicians who left the PHS to return to private practice carried with them an increased awareness of the importance of public health and the role of federal agencies in preventing the spread of diseases.[14]

Within the world of private medicine and day-to-day medical care, radical changes were also occurring. Throughout the 1960s and 1970s, employer-based health insurance remained the norm for most Americans. But the birth of Medicaid and Medicare in 1965 meant that the federal government now had a direct hand in the medical treatment of millions of Americans.[15] Two other federally funded health care programs, the Indian Health Service and the Veterans Administration, also expanded rapidly during this period. By the late 1960s, as millions of Americans began receiving health care directly funded by the American government, reformers began to agitate for a further expansion of federal health care to cover all Americans. Attempts to nationalize health insurance failed, but the reform movement that emerged during this period shaped many federal officials' approach to public health. In fact, so many HEW officials believed that a coherent and fully funded national health care system would soon be implemented that they often proposed public health initiatives with this assumption in mind.

The lure of a federally funded form of health insurance was especially appealing during this period as both physicians and the general public had tremendous confidence in the medical profession's ability to cure and even eradicate diseases. To some degree this confidence seemed justified, as a series of PHS-sponsored campaigns successfully controlled polio, eradicated smallpox, prevented tooth decay by fluoridating the nation's drinking water, and sharply limited the impact of environmental dangers. While the surgeon general, William Stewart, may not have made the claim often attributed to him that the age of infectious disease was ending, this belief did shape the actions of the diverse medical professionals whom he directly supervised in the Public Health Service.[16]

Like smallpox and polio, sexual ignorance, illegitimate pregnancy, and venereal disease were seen by the public health community as very solvable problems. But this optimism also had its downside. The government's overwhelming confidence in its ability to eradicate disease translated into a tendency to underestimate the complex threat posed by Americans' ignorance about sexuality. Looking back at the period from the vantage of 2005, former Surgeon General Jesse Steinfeld remembered that the Public Health Service did not view venereal disease as a significant problem because "we did have therapies for syphilis and gonorrhea." Unwanted pregnancies were also viewed differently

than they had been in the past because the advent of the birth control pill promised to make unwanted pregnancies obsolete. Similarly, "other advances which
made the risk [associated with] pregnancy much less" meant that the PHS, or at
least its leaders, were more inclined to view smallpox, polio, and other diseases
as greater threats than unplanned or difficult pregnancies.[17]

Although the head of the Public Health Service downgraded the threat posed
by sexual ignorance, rank-and-file members of the Service remained concerned
about the public's lack of sexual knowledge. Venereal disease, as the CDC well
knew, dogged many communities, while illegitimate births were on the rise, especially in poor areas. Outside the narrow government enclaves in Washington
and the CDC in Atlanta, many Americans, particularly those who viewed with
alarm the changing sexual behavior of their fellow citizens, also saw these issues
as significant problems. Reflecting these concerns, the popular press spawned
an increasing number of articles with titles such as "Sex Education: How Much?
How Soon?" and "What Kids Still Don't Know about Sex."[18]

In response to this pressure, federal officials demanded an extremely comprehensive sex education campaign. As with previous campaigns, this new program promised to teach Americans "everything they always wanted to know
about sex but were afraid to ask." But the materials produced during this period
once again took a scattershot approach to the problem. Programs and initiatives
came from a variety of agencies within the federal government, and limited in-
teraction between these agencies meant that the program that emerged lacked
a coherent focus. Compounding these problems was a series of internal turf battles within the Public Health Service. By the late 1960s these battles had resulted in a restructuring of the PHS, one that splintered the organization and
sharply limited the powers of the surgeon general.

Diseases and Unwanted Children

"Did your old man ever take you into the bedroom and give you the old pep
talk? About women and diseases?" The answer was a no-brainer: "My dad never
told me a thing." For fifteen-year-old Arthur, as for many of his peers, ignorance was a sure path to bliss, but the bliss was only temporary. When his girl-
friend became pregnant, Arthur found himself at a loss. Where could he and
Janet go for advice? What were their options? *Were* there any options?

A fictional creation of the playwrights James Leo Herlihy and William
Noble, Arthur was the grandchild of George Dupont, the hero of Upton Sin-

clair's early-twentieth-century play *Damaged Goods*. Like Arthur, George had been a victim of his parents' refusal to educate him about sex. But in 1913 George's sexual ignorance led him to contract venereal disease. By the mid-twentieth century, with penicillin readily available, the nation's concerns about sexual ignorance had shifted. Arthur's ignorance led not to disease but to an unwanted pregnancy.[19]

Out-of-wedlock pregnancies, or illegitimate births, as they were then termed, had long been a concern of the Public Health Service. By the 1960s and 1970s, as birth control methods dramatically improved, public health experts began to reassess the term *unwanted pregnancy*. By the late 1960s,the phrase referred not only to all illegitimate births but also to any unplanned birth. Reflecting the common prejudices of the day, PHS officials insisted that the children of unplanned pregnancies were more likely to endure physical abuse and neglect than their "wanted" peers. This view eerily paralleled the Public Health Service's early-twentieth-century arguments about the high costs of caring for children whose parents inadvertently infected them with venereal disease. At that time, public health experts had declared that the nation could ill afford the damaged children who were the offspring of sexually diseased parents.[20]

The costs of unwanted offspring were not defined in simply financial terms. Beginning in the late 1950s, public health experts both in and outside the federal government had argued that the failure to implement a comprehensive family-planning program would cause a severe population crisis while putting extreme pressure on limited resources. This crisis would, it was believed, cause severe global famines as well as shortages of oil. Throughout the 1960s and into the 1970s, the federal government and private foundations alike publicized this belief. By the late 1960s, concerns about overpopulation had reached such levels that novels and films now overwhelmingly depicted a bleak future society in which overpopulation leads to cannibalism *(Soylent Green)*, mass homicide *(Quality of Mercy)*, and mass executions *(Logan's Run)*. Women's magazines, such as *Redbook*, *McCalls*, and *Parents' Magazine*, refrained from the sensationalism of science fiction, but they did publish repeated articles warning of a population explosion. All of this publicity convinced Americans that overpopulation was one of the greatest threats facing mankind, and by the late 1960s most people were willing to support federal initiatives to deal with these problems. In 1970, pressure from both the public health community and the general public led to the passage of the Family Planning Services and Population Research Act. The Act "created two new agencies with HEW, the National Center for Population and Family Planning under the direct supervision of the assistant secretary for health and scientific affairs and the National Center for Planning Services."[21] Linking the problems caused by rapid urbanization and pollution to fears that the welfare rolls were growing, Senator Joseph Tydings, a Democrat from Maryland, summed up the sentiments of many of his fellow Americans, both Republicans and Democrats. "Any realistic campaign to eliminate poverty in America must," Tydings maintained, "include programs that make family planning information and services available on a voluntary basis."[22]

Tackling the issue of family planning directly would require teaching men and women, boys and girls, about contraception. The government, which had always seen the battle against disease as its central goal, would now embark on a battle against unwanted pregnancy, a much less clearly defined battle than the fight against a biological disease. As the government's role shifted, the nation's citizens would have to accept a new understanding of the role the government could or should play in assisting Americans to plan their families. Encouraging Americans to rethink both their notions of public health and the role of the government would be a monumental task. Yet within the history of the federal government, there was a strong precedent for this new focus on family planning. Federal officials, both in and outside the Public Health Service, had always recognized a strong connection between poverty and disease. By casting the battle against unwanted pregnancy as both part of their own tradition of fighting disease and as a response to Johnson's War on Poverty, many officials believed, the birth rate among teenagers and unmarried women, along with rates of venereal disease, would drop to all-time lows.

In many ways this optimism made sense. The early 1960s had witnessed "a substantial amount of research on both reproduction and birth control."[23] True, the early 1960s had witnessed a substantial jump in the birth rate among teens, but the CDC was carefully tracking these numbers in an attempt to contain them. Moreover, as even the most zealous of the Public Health Service's critics knew, rising rates of teen pregnancy were as much a result of the demographic bulge caused by millions of baby boomers becoming adolescents as they were a result of a broader social shift in sexual behavior that was caused, in turn, by a larger population of adolescents.[24] But while the PHS acknowledged the baby boom's complex impact on the rates of illegitimate pregnancy, federal officials were reluctant to rely on easy excuses. Instead of shrugging off the problem, PHS officials advocated a variety of aggressive initiatives, including educational programs, to forestall or limit any future rise in teenage pregnancies.

One of the most aggressive of these measures was the implementation of Title X. Title X had been passed as part of the Family Planning Services and Population Research Act, which had enabled the federal government to "assist in making comprehensive family planning services readily available to all persons desiring such services."[25] Basically, Title X ensured that all Americans, regardless of their income, could obtain access to family-planning services and contraception. Eight years after its implementation, the Act was amended to place special emphasis on preventing unwanted pregnancies among adolescents. Although the focus of Title X was always on providing direct family-planning services, the act had repercussions for sex education, as many women and teenagers received crucial information and education on human sexuality while receiving care related to family planning.

Even as the Public Health Service became more aggressive in fighting unwanted pregnancy, federal officials remained optimistic about the government's ability to eradicate syphilis. As late as 1965 the Service was predicting that education and treatment would eradicate the disease by 1972. Improved testing for syphilis combined with better and more extensive epidemiological studies of outbreaks boded well for this effort, as did the development and implementation of a "comprehensive educational program to reach the general public and . . . professional personnel." By 1965 the educational program had reached a variety of urban communities, including several cities that had been at the forefront of previous educational campaigns. Promising as this new approach to sex education was, this focus on urban areas tended to neglect rural areas, which were, despite the stereotype of the idyllic small town, hardly free from venereal disease.[26]

Looking back at the 1960s from the vantage of 1969, federal officials must have breathed a sigh of relief. During the preceding decade the Public Health Service had made remarkable gains in identifying and moving to control new and growing problems associated with venereal diseases and unwanted pregnancies. Yet even as the PHS made these gains, Americans remained reluctant to embrace aggressive and candid programs promoting sex education. As Robert Finch, the secretary of HEW, well knew, the government's successes in this field stemmed from the fact that the PHS and HEW had "played a hypocritical game for many years" by creating family-planning and sex education programs that were then "obscure[d] . . . with other names." But now a different tactic, one employing a new openness, was needed. And "having just about run out of people we can offend," as Finch wryly put it, the government was finally prepared to launch what it believed would be a truly comprehensive sex education campaign.[27]

But federal officials remained constrained by their concerns about offending the more conservative segments of American society. This fear would continue, as it always had, to plague federally funded efforts to promote sexual literacy. The issue of birth control, as Finch and others would discover, would prove to be especially complex and controversial in the decades that followed. Venereal disease would in many ways be less controversial, but the threat caused by sexually transmitted diseases would, as all Americans now know, experience only a temporary lull during this period.

The Total Picture

When a new task force was formed in 1969 to address the problem of preventative medicine, federal officials foresaw few of these problems. Instead, committee members believed that after decades of dithering, Americans were finally willing to confront and discuss "the whole problem of human reproduction" as never before. The issues of "conception/contraception, defect/death, wanted/unwanted [children], and even the problem of postnatal infant mortality as a consequence of disease or the battered child," would now move to the forefront of public health. One member of the federally appointed task force even went so far as to argue that the time had come for PHS and HEW officials to "look at the total picture and see where abortion fits in."[28] This call to include abortion in the broader discussion of sex education reflected public health experts' belief that this procedure would soon be legalized in all American states.

By the 1960s, abortion had a long history in America. In the two and a half centuries following the first European settlement in North America, poor understanding of contraception had made abortion a necessity for many couples who needed to limit their families. Reflecting longstanding European attitudes toward abortion, the practice had in fact been legal in most states. Beginning in the mid-nineteenth century, however, states rushed to ban the procedure. There were multiple reasons behind this impetus to ban abortion, but paramount among them was educated physicians' fear that abortionists, many of whom were women, were performing a procedure that was difficult to perform safely. Physicians, who were struggling to establish themselves as the nation's principal medical practitioners, also resented the way in which abortionists added to the competition for patients. By making abortion illegal, many physicians believed that they could both prohibit a dangerous and difficult procedure and advance their own profession. Making abortion illegal did not prevent women from seeking out practitioners who would perform the procedure. And throughout the early twentieth century, "in many local communities, the local abortion practitioner's name and address were well-known." Additionally, an "unwritten law prevailed between law enforcement and practitioners: no deaths, no prosecution."[29]

During the postwar period, this lax approach to abortion shifted as American culture came to place an emphasis on domesticity and motherhood. White women, particularly single white women, who became pregnant during this era were now encouraged to carry the fetus to term and then give the child up for adoption. Single African-American women, whose babies lacked value in the adoption market, were also encouraged to carry the fetus to term, but they were often encouraged to keep and raise the child, themselves. Unlike white women, African-American women who became pregnant out of wedlock were also often encouraged to become sterilized after an unwanted pregnancy.[30] This draconian approach to unwanted pregnancy ultimately sparked a backlash; increasingly, the general public, women, and medical practitioners began to argue that a woman had the right to determine whether she would carry a pregnancy to term. In 1970 two attorneys represented Norma L. McCorvey (Jane Roe), who had become pregnant as a result of a rape. The case moved to the Supreme Court, where it was determined that the illegalization of abortion violated, among other things, a constitutional right to privacy. The case impacted forty-six states, all of which had laws restricting abortion.

Despite this shift in the law, the Public Health Service continued to be wary of proposing abortion as a means to combat unwanted pregnancy in the decades following *Roe v. Wade*. The reasons for this reluctance were fairly clear. Transcripts from meetings in the late 1960s indicate that many public health experts and federal officials worried that they would be associated with advocating abortions solely or even primarily for poor or minority women. Given the history of the Public Health Service's role in the Tuskegee Syphilis Experiment as well as its role in encouraging African-American women to be sterilized, this caution was understandable. Although it was not widely promoted, abortion did, however, remain very much a part of the discussion about federally funded sex education efforts during this period.[31]

PHS and HEW officials may have been ill prepared to tackle abortion in their sex education campaign, but they were willing to tackle other equally difficult issues. David Sencer, the director of the CDC, saw the biggest problem facing any sex education campaign as the "question of how . . . you keep . . . communities continually interested" in syphilis and gonorrhea, especially when disease rates were declining. Public health experts overwhelmingly agreed with Sencer's concerns. However, they were quick to point out that many lower socioeconomic groups had viewed rising rates of venereal disease with little concern. Any action taken by the government, Sencer's opponents argued, needed first to address the very serious problems that existed in communities that were already suffering from high rates of venereal disease. Only then could the government hope to create a program that would sustain motivation in the face of declining disease rates. While federal officials might be excused for dodging such a difficult issue, this approach meant that the government would continue to follow the approach it had always taken: rushing in to deal with venereal disease when the rates of these diseases soared while postponing any serious attempt to create a program that would keep communities actively engaged in the fight against venereal disease. A similar view shaped the government's battle against teen and unwanted pregnancies. Again, this meant there was little hope that the government would be able to initiate a long-term plan to control or limit unwanted pregnancies.[32]

Overall, the government's response to this problem was both conservative and reflective of the times. Middle-class practitioners were urged to take a back seat and allow community activists to assume a larger role in both educating communities and providing them with contraceptives and medical assistance. In the words of one public health expert, "Without citizen participation these programs cannot be successful."[33] Citizen participation included enabling members of different communities to participate directly in the creation and implementation of sex education and family-planning programs. It also meant depicting ethnic minorities on all educational pamphlets and other materials released by HEW. In advocating this approach, the Public Health Service was unknowingly continuing earlier policies. In 1918, when the PHS had launched its first sex education campaign, citizen participation had been seen as central to its success. Segregation, combined with racial prejudices, had also led the PHS to create separate pamphlets featuring minorities that were intended for distribution in minority communities. These older pamphlets had, of course, endorsed racial and ethnic stereotypes, but they had been groundbreaking in that they attempted to address the specific concerns of minority groups.[34]

Unfortunately, even as the federal government reassessed its approach to minority sex education, new problems had come to the fore. Many African-American leaders, including Martin Luther King, endorsed the federal government's call to use family planning as a means of controlling poverty, but others were more suspicious. Radical revolutionary groups such as the Black Panthers and the Black Muslims harshly condemned the government's family-planning initiatives and any corresponding sex education programs, seeing in them evidence of federally sponsored "black genocide." For those who may have questioned this sweeping condemnation of federal policies, both the Tuskegee Syphilis Experiment and the government's sterilization policies appeared to provide ample evidence of government animosity toward African Americans. Not all African Americans endorsed this view, of course. Responses to federally sponsored family planning initiatives often split along class lines, with middle-class African Americans endorsing these measures while working-class and poor African Americans were more resistant to these efforts. Attitudes toward family planning also split along gender lines. African-American women often strongly advocated the use of family planning, but African-American men, especially those who were already suspicious of the federal government, saw these efforts in a negative light. The government's overt targeting of minority communities and the justified suspicion with which many African Americans viewed the federal government meant that sex education programs would continue to encounter difficulties in minority communities throughout this period.

Despite both these tensions and the suspicion with which many African Americans viewed white public health experts, federal officials did not believe that public health and community activists needed to be members of the minority groups they were trying to reach. Pointing out that "undergraduate students in colleges and universities have [recently] confronted society and higher education . . . [on the subject of] racism, free speech . . . peace, [and] participation in decision making," the government called for an "alliance between the new students and the older generations in control of public affairs." The greatest activism would be found among students of medicine and dentistry, who would endorse the belief that "health and health services are a right" and who would work to further this right among diverse populations.[35]

The belief that both citizen partnerships and links to community activists were crucial to the success of sex education programs stemmed from the supposition that people needed to be invested in a sex education program if it were to succeed. But this technique was also highly expedient. Partnerships with citizen organizations enabled the government to operate programs cheaply using both funds and manpower from local communities. Historically this approach had produced mixed results. Organizations that shared the government's commitment to sex education tended to provide excellent support while organizations that were not deeply committed to the government's programs had often provided little to none. In the latter case some of the government's sex education programs had begun to founder even before they were fully established. Lacking any information about this history of citizen partnerships, public health experts strongly endorsed the use of these partnerships in 1969 with little or no debate over the benefits and drawbacks inherent in this type of approach. Ironically, in advocating the use of partnerships, government officials were not only repeating past mistakes, they were also contributing to an existing and widely recognized problem in the structure of the American health care system: the use of public-private partnerships.

In a 1968 report to the president, Wilbur Cohen, then secretary of HEW, had pointed out that "the American system of health care, research, education, and disease prevention is a mosaic of private and public efforts." Cohen had actually called for the federal government to assume control of state efforts to promote public health as well as efforts organized by private and nonprofit health organizations. He believed that he had taken steps to assure that this would occur. However, the changes Cohen advocated were minor, and the government's ability to direct nationwide initiatives remained sharply limited. As early as 1969, public health experts were well aware that the nation's piecemeal approach to public health and health care had already led to serious deficiencies in most government-sponsored programs. Some public health experts expressed concern that this piecemeal approach to health care would hamper any effective and consistent nationwide plan for sex education.[36]

High Ideals, Harsh Realities

The government's reliance on community-level sex education arrangements did not mean that the Public Health Service abandoned or even surrendered control of sex education programs completely during the 1970s. The PHS reissued and updated several sex education pamphlets during this period. It also created new materials for teenagers and adults.

Among the pamphlets the Public Health Service updated and rereleased was *Strictly for Teenagers: Some Facts about Venereal Disease*. When first released in the 1960s, *Strictly for Teenagers* called upon teenagers to "talk frankly about venereal disease." The original pamphlet showed teenagers earnestly engaging in activities deemed appropriate for teenagers in the 1960s. The cover of the 1964 pamphlet featured clean-cut adolescents wearing button-down shirts and smocked dresses earnestly peering through microscopes and taking diligent notes. Within the pamphlet, teenagers are shown on a date. Although the boy has his arm on the back of his date's chair, the most stimulating elements portrayed are the caffeinated sodas. The rereleased pamphlet from the early 1970s shows something quite different. The clean-cut adolescents from the soda shop have been transformed into bell-bottomed teens speeding off to a date on a motorcycle. The girl, wearing a sleeveless shirt that exposes her neck, clutches her date's waist with her pelvis pushed against his body. Compared with his clean-cut counterpart in the pamphlet from the 1960s, the boy on the motorcycle looks older. He wears a leather or jeans jacket, clothes often associated with disaffected youth and rebellion, and his face is hidden behind dark sunglasses. These teens, unlike those in the soda shop, seem much more likely to be heading off to engage in sexual intercourse.

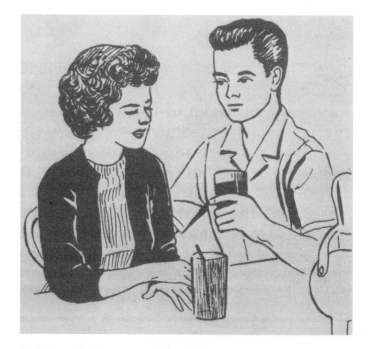

It seems unlikely that this earnest conversation in a soda shop will wind up with a visit to a bedroom. *Strictly for Teenagers* (1964). Department of Health and Human Services.

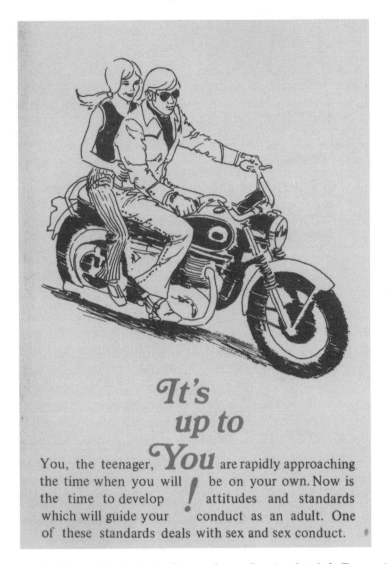

It's
up to
You

You, the teenager, are rapidly approaching the time when you will *!* be on your own. Now is the time to develop attitudes and standards which will guide your conduct as an adult. One of these standards deals with sex and sex conduct.

Up to no good? A boy and his date head off in an unknown direction. *Strictly for Teenagers* (1971). Department of Health and Human Services.

While the Public Health Service was willing to update the imagery in its sex education materials to reflect the reality of teens having sex, it saw little need to update the text. Did federal officials swallow the naive belief, stated in both 1964 and 1971, that "the high ideals of most teenagers help rule out the possibility of their contracting venereal disease"?[37] PHS officials did seem earnestly to believe in the same message that they had been touting since the 1920s. Fundamentally, the PHS continued to assume that teens could be dissuaded from sexual experimentation and that American parents were not yet prepared for an overt acknowledgment that their teenage children were sexually active.

In many ways the Public Health Service was right in making this assessment. Television, which had now become one of the best monitors of American culture simply by virtue of its widespread popularity and its limited number of channels, provides perhaps the best insight into Americans' conservative views on sexual behavior. On the surface, television shows from this period appear to endorse a more liberal approach to sex. The 1970s in particular have been notoriously characterized as the age of "jiggle-television," with shows such as *Charlie's Angels* and *Three's Company* aired during prime time to the nation's adolescents and adults. But even as these shows exploited the "jiggle factor," Americans remained in denial about the consequences of so much "jiggle." With a few notable exceptions, the real and very complex issues of unwanted pregnancy, venereal disease, and premarital sex were almost always sidelined or, at best, treated superficially by this medium. *Family*, one of the more popular shows, which ran between 1976 and 1980, was typical in this regard. The show's writers were willing to acknowledge that teens engaged in sex, but they kept on the safe side by having the show's wildly popular teen star Kristy McNichol expressly opt *not* to have sex.[38] Those shows that did have teens engage in sex and that did candidly discuss venereal disease and teen pregnancies, such as *James at Fifteen/Sixteen*, sparked controversies and experienced relatively short lives as a result.[39]

But outside the safety of television's idyllic suburbs, the Public Health Service had only to look at rising rates of venereal disease and teenage pregnancy to know that teens were engaging in sex. By 1977 the PHS was forced to ask Americans if teenage pregnancy really was "someone else's problem." And just as it had taken a tentative step forward in the 1930s when it released a pamphlet that frankly explained how barrier methods could prevent venereal disease, the government now took a radical step forward by releasing another groundbreaking pamphlet, *Teenage Pregnancy: Everyone's Problem.*

Insisting that "we can make sure that there is a place where sexually active teenage boys and girls can receive reliable information," the pamphlet detailed six methods by which teens could prevent pregnancy. Among these techniques were the pill, the IUD, the diaphragm, the condom, foam, and "natural meth-ods" such as the rhythm method. Including the last of these methods was un-doubtedly done with an eye to appeasing the nation's most conservative ele-ments. But in providing information about the rhythm method, the Public Health Service was not prepared to throw caution completely to the wind. Nat-ural methods, the pamphlet maintained, are effective only when the "woman and her partner fully understand them." This caveat was accompanied by a warning that the method worked best when the woman had regular menstrual cycles. While it is unclear how many teenagers would have taken the first part of this warning seriously, the issue of regular periods may have led some teenagers to reconsider this method. As many teenage girls know, a teenager's menstrual cycles are often irregular.

Teenage Pregnancy went a step beyond simply providing teenagers with hon-est and frank discussions of contraception. The pamphlet also discussed abor-tion and the need for teenage girls to have access to safe and inexpensive abor-tions. However, even as the Public Health Service provided information on obtaining abortions to young women (as was their legal right), it was still cau-tious about the use of abortions. The pamphlet did not overtly condemn women who had abortions or overtly discourage women from seeking them. However, it did stress that "some doctors think that abortions, or particularly repeated abortions in very young girls, may impair their health and ability to have chil-dren later." This caution was in many ways similar to the more general cautions the PHS had issued regarding teenagers carrying a pregnancy to term. Having a child while a teenager, the PHS insisted, may negatively impact a young mother's "ability to function in a productive way later in life and it may help ex-plain the relatively high rate of suicide among older women who experienced a pregnancy in their teens."[40]

How widely *Teenage Pregnancy: Everyone's Problem* was circulated is unclear. As was typical with all of the government's educational campaigns, Americans had to request the pamphlet directly from the Public Health Service. While studies have indicated that many Americans do request medical pamphlets pub-lished by the government and private organizations, this distribution approach may have meant that those who read the pamphlets were precisely those in least need of advice. All of this meant that the Public Health Service's efforts, even at their most innovative, failed to reach many of the Americans who wanted and needed comprehensive sex education.

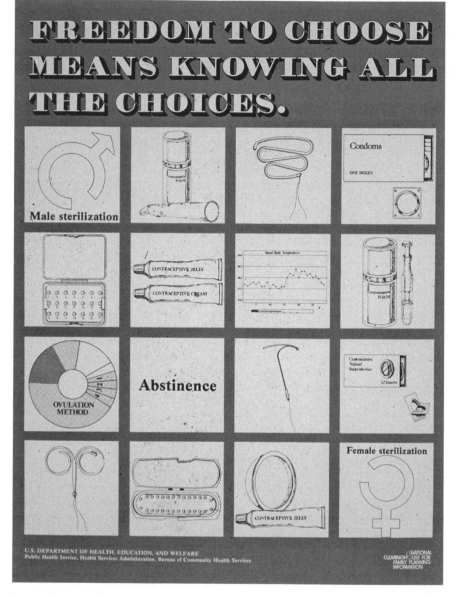

Posters also provided Americans with comprehensive information about birth control methods (ca. 1970s). Department of Health and Human Services.

New Programs and the Possibility of a New Future

The creation and implementation of Medicaid and Medicare in 1965 "clearly insure[d] that the Federal health effort better serve[d] the health needs of the American people," but Public Health Service officers remained uncertain as to how these new programs could benefit the fight against sexually transmitted diseases or the push to improve Americans' understanding of family planning.[41]

Even the most optimistic government experts found it difficult to believe that the government's new entitlement programs would immediately or directly benefit educational programs to improve public health. At best, experts saw Medicaid and Medicare as presaging broader changes that would completely reshape the American health care system over the next ten years. These changes would, public health experts believed, gradually unfold during the 1970s, opening up new streams of funding for both better health care and more comprehensive programs in preventive medicine. Sex education, which fell under the rubric of preventive medicine, would benefit from these trends. But if public health experts were optimistic about the potential of Medicaid and Medicare to improve preventive medicine in general, they also worried that these initiatives would create serious difficulties for public health campaigns in the short term. One senior public health expert summed up the problem by cautioning that these new programs "simultaneously impose[d] a greatly increased and changed demand on already overtaxed health resources."[42]

As was always true with government public health initiatives, funding, especially guaranteed funding, was an uncertainty. One tack the Public Health Service tried was to link its own calls for improved sex education to broader government initiatives. In 1970, for example, the PHS pushed for the 1970 White House Conference on Children and Youth to address sex education. Provided with a budget of about $2.8 million (1960s dollars), the Conference would attract the attention of the nation's leading experts in public health, including those on a state and local level. It also had the potential to educate the mainstream press and laypeople on the benefits of sex education programs. But as the PHS discovered, to its cost, issues relating to "family planning and sex education" were easily lost in the broader discussion of the needs of children and adolescents.[43]

By the early and mid-1970s, even as the Public Health Service initiated a new program on sex education and made remarkable strides forward with pamphlets such as *Teenage Pregnancy: Everyone's Problem*, funding for sex education was being cut. The Nixon, Ford, and Carter administrations' focus on controlling inflation led to a moratorium on new projects. Existing programs, especially sex education programs, were strangled while other proposed projects were stillborn. The failure to invest in preventive sexual health programs had extremely high costs. In his study of venereal disease in America, Allan Brandt has pointed out that the costs of treating sexually transmitted diseases in the 1970s far outstripped federal spending on programs aimed at controlling these diseases. While the costs of unwanted pregnancies are more difficult to determine, the rapid rise in teenage pregnancies during this period also indicates that the government's failure to invest in comprehensive and aggressive sex education during this period did little to save money in the long run.[44]

This lack of funding was not the only impediment confronting federal officials as they wrestled with the issue of sex education. During the 1960s and 1970s, American society did not undergo the monumental transformations that HEW and PHS officials had hoped would occur. Surgeon General Jesse Steinfeld had warned his fellow public health experts that "medical education is by its very nature a conservative thing."[45] And indeed, most medical students did not become activists, demanding that all Americans receive access to preventive medicine and information on the prevention of sexually transmitted diseases. Obviously, in believing that the changes in the American health care system would be implemented, even demanded, by student activists, the Public Health Service and HEW had counted too much on the power and durability of student activism. During the 1970s, as student activism declined, the younger generation, which public health experts had rather naively believed would be so eager to implement broad sweeping changes in preventive medicine and sex education, failed to take up the cause of reform.

In many ways this failure could have been predicted. Medical students' apathy toward sex education campaigns stemmed in part from the fact that "about two thirds of all medical schools do not have departments of preventive medicine."[46] To influence the younger generation's understanding of preventive care and public health education, the committee needed to change the curriculum offered in the nation's medical schools. This was not a challenge they were willing to undertake at that time.

The government's biggest failure, however, stemmed from its inability to articulate a clear and concise goal. Containing sexually transmitted diseases was one important goal. But HEW and PHS officials also considered abortion, the rising numbers of illegitimate births among the nation's many teenagers, the inability of many married women to understand and use contraceptives effectively, and the prevalence of what they called "battered child syndrome" among families where children were unwanted and/or unplanned to be serious problems. Understanding and addressing just one of these concerns would have necessitated that public health experts take up and resolve a range of highly complex issues, not the least of which was how to reach every American. Ultimately this lack of a unified and coherent message may have doomed the Public Health Service's attempt to promote sexual health among Americans during the 1960s and 1970s, just as it had doomed previous attempts in the preceding decades.

TELLING IT LIKE IT IS
1981–1988

It's done in plain language, it's done at a 12- to 13-year-old
reading level, it doesn't mince words, yet it is in good taste
and stresses proper behavior, values and responsibilities.

OTIS BOWEN, SECRETARY OF HEALTH
AND HUMAN SERVICES, 1988

You should wear a condom from start to finish.

SURGEON GENERAL C. EVERETT KOOP, 1988

I t began slowly. AIDS, C. Everett Koop said, "entered the consciousness of
the Public Health Service rather quietly, rather gradually, and with almost
no fanfare at all."[1] In early June of 1981, PHS staffers learned that five homosexual males had developed an extremely rare disease, *Pneumocystis carinni*
pneumonia (PCP). Over the course of the summer more reports of individuals
suffering from PCP began to trickle in. By the early fall, Anthony Fauci, a leading researcher in immunology at the National Institutes of Health, began "to
get a little worried thinking that this might be the emergence of a new disease."
"I started," he said, "to get goose pimples." Almost from the onset, researchers
began to suspect that the disease might be transmitted by blood and sex, an especially worrisome proposition, as this type of transmission meant that the disease would not remain confined to a small population. After all, sex, as Fauci
drily remarked, "is a universal thing," meaning that the spread of the disease
among a wider population was just a matter of time.[2]

That summer, as public health experts at the Centers for Disease Control
(CDC) and the National Institutes of Health (NIH) began to explore the possibility of a new disease, the national media focused not on the emerging public health crisis but rather on a more heated debate unfolding in Congress: the
confirmation of a new surgeon general for the U.S. Public Health Service.
C. Everett Koop, a pediatrician from Philadelphia, had been tapped by Presi-

dent Ronald Reagan to serve in the nation's highest position in the field of public health. Koop's appointment quickly became mired in controversy. According to Senator Ted Kennedy, the controversy was about Dr. Koop's lack of "experience in public health, in programs emphasizing the prevention of disease and the health needs of the population as a whole."[3] But as the medical journal *Hospital Practice* pointed out, the causes behind the controversy were more complex: "Koop was also a fundamentalist Christian and his appointment was taken as a signal that the administration [wanted] . . . to reverse the legalization of abortion [which had been] achieved with *Roe v. Wade*."[4] Koop's nomination quickly became so problematic that the American Public Health Association, the oldest and largest professional public health society in the United States, publicly "broke its one hundred year tradition of silence on Presidential nominees for surgeon general and vigorously opposed the nomination of Dr. Koop."[5]

While the storm that swirled around his nomination was political in nature, Koop's qualifications were more problematic than his supporters were prepared to admit. Senator Jesse Helms might rail against both "stereotypes about anti-abortionists" and unfair "allegations of religious fanaticism and antiwoman attitudes," but Koop's opponents had strong grounds for questioning his qualifications for the nation's highest position in public health. As Koop admitted in an interview several years later, "I never saw myself as a person who was involved in public health, [until] . . . I came to Washington and had to justify the fact that I thought I could be the Surgeon General of the Public Health Service." Koop's knowledge of public health was limited to one course he had taken in medical school decades previously.[6] In this respect his nomination for surgeon general was unique. With the exception of Julius Richmond, who had at least spent several decades in the field of public health, all previous surgeons general had been drawn from the ranks of the Public Health Service.

Supporters who insisted that "so much of the hostility to[ward] Koop" stemmed from factors unrelated to public health were not completely off the mark, however. Koop's opponents included a range of groups outside the field of public health, groups whose main concerns revolved around his opposition to abortion or, more simply, his background as an evangelical Christian. The American Association of University Women, the National Organization of Women, the B'nai B'rith Women, and a variety of other organizations opposing Koop were more concerned about his opposition to abortion than his lack of experience in the field of public health. And given the limited understanding of AIDS in the fall of 1981, it seems likely that organizations such as the National Gay Health Coalition and the United Presbyterian Church, which went on record as opposing the nomination, were more concerned about Koop's background as an evangelical than his limited knowledge of public health.

All of this opposition meant a contentious confirmation hearing. Yet despite the heated tenor of the debate, Koop was ultimately confirmed, with a vote of 64 to 28 in the Senate. The press and Koop himself believed that the controversy had ended, but the truth, of course, was that it had barely begun.

As surgeon general, Koop would come to embody the Public Health Service as no previous surgeon general had. During his eight-year tenure as head of the Public Health Service, Koop's public calls for better sex education, combined with his attacks on the tobacco industry, would make him a lightning rod for a diverse range of forces in American society.[7]

Brave New World

When C. Everett Koop became surgeon general, he became the head of an agency in flux. During his tenure the Public Health Service would close the hospitals that had been at the center of the Service for almost two hundred years, thereby radically transforming the overall mission of the agency. The Commissioned Corps, the ranked officer corps of the PHS, would come under attack. The arrival on U.S. shores of Cuban refugees as Koop was being vetted for the post would threaten to import serious diseases such as hepatitis, tuberculosis, and leprosy. More traditional problems, such as increases in the numbers of teenagers who became pregnant or infected with syphilis and gonorrhea, would spark heated and very public debates about the goals and structure of sex education. But the advent of AIDS would do the most to transform the ways in which the American public viewed infectious diseases, public health, and sex education.

Knowing little about the agency's complex history in developing sex education programs, Koop was wildly optimistic about what he would be able to accomplish in the battle against teenage pregnancy and sexually transmitted diseases, specifically AIDS. Knowing even less about the heated nature of Washington politics, Koop also assumed that the administration would allow him to advocate sex education programs in any form he deemed appropriate. These assumptions turned out to be wrong. For the first five and a half years of his tenure, Surgeon General Koop was forbidden to speak publicly on AIDS. He was also not invited to join the high-level PHS task force that was created to deal with the many different facets of the growing epidemic. This marginalization of the head of the Public Health Service meant that the PHS came to be seen as indifferent to the AIDS epidemic, at least during the early 1980s.

Battling for and against Sex Education

Seventeen-year-old Glen Bond did not know much about sex. "I want a response that gets down to basics," he told a reporter in 1981. "I want the main definition instead of someone just saying 'Um, um, um.'" For Glen, the best source of information was his friends. That they might not know more than he did was irrelevant; the plain fact was that he was more comfortable asking them. But there were, as Glen well knew, better sources for sex education.[8]

Reflecting the private-public mosaic that characterizes American health care in general, both public and private institutions had long been at the forefront of providing Americans with frank, unbiased, and comprehensive information about sex, sexually transmitted diseases, and reproduction. Freed from the need to please a diverse electorate, private organizations such as Planned Parenthood and the Sexuality Information and Education Council of the United States (SIECUS) along with research organizations such as the Alan Guttmacher Institute had grown tremendously during the 1970s. By 1980 many Americans viewed these institutions, not the federal government, as providing the best and most comprehensive form of sex education available in the United States. However, state and local governments as well as the federal government still remained central players in the battle for sexual literacy during this period. The Public Health Service in particular continued to issue educational pamphlets on sex, and PHS agencies continued to work to address the many questions about sex that Glen Bond and other teenagers had.[9] Additionally, because the federal government worked so closely with private organizations, providing them with grants and other forms of funding, these organizations often reflected the views of federal officials.

By the mid-1980s, growing numbers of teens had become sexually active. Rates of venereal disease and teenage pregnancy had also risen significantly, making the issue of sex education increasingly urgent. But here, sex education experts, both in and outside the government, found themselves stymied.

Thirteen years before Glen began looking for answers about his questions on sex, a major battle over sex education had erupted in the Anaheim, California, school district. That year Eleanor Howe, who had several children in the district, launched an all-out attack on the Family and Sex Life Education program used in the Anaheim public schools. Howe represented a minority view in her community, and her allegations against the nation's sex education programs were often misleading, if not patently untrue. Nevertheless, she was able to garner tremendous support by tapping into Americans' general uneasiness with sex education and their discomfort with the more extreme aspects of the sexual revolution. Within a few years Howe had taken her movement national. Across the United States, city council meetings became increasingly contentious as opponents and supporters of sex education clashed. Teachers, nurses, and public health experts were forced to defend themselves against a rash of accusations, and local officials discovered, often to their dismay, that their views on sex education could mean the difference between defeat and victory at the ballot box.[10]

In many ways Howe's success in battling sex education reflected a broader shift in American politics, the rise of what has often been called the Christian or Religious Right. While it is possible to trace the origins of the Christian Right back to the early twentieth century, the emergence of this movement in its modern form was rooted in the changes that had occurred in the 1960s and early 1970s. Responding to the civil rights movement, the Vietnam War, the women's movement, the sexual revolution, the banning of prayer in schools, the threat of communism, and the legalization of abortion, conservative Christians rallied around charismatic figures such as Pat Robertson, Jerry Falwell, and Phyllis Schlafly during the late 1960s and early 1970s.

From its beginning the Christian Right was an uneasy coalition of diverse groups. Jerry Falwell, who headed one of the leading organizations associated with the Christian Right, the Moral Majority, saw his group as a "political organization, not a religious one."[11] Falwell's group included not only fundamentalists (those who believed in a literal interpretation of the Bible) but also evangelicals (those who testified to a personal faith). Because the dividing line between fundamentalists and evangelicals is a fine one, and because many Protestants consider themselves to be both fundamentalists and evangelicals, the political unification of these two groups was not surprising. But the Moral Majority and later, the Christian Coalition, also attracted those outside the Protestant community. Since the late 1960s, Catholics, Orthodox Jews, Mormons, and even secularists have either overtly joined forces with this predominantly Protestant movement or developed parallel and very similar organizations. By the mid-1970s the Christian Right—or, to use a better term, the

Religious Right—had become fully engaged in what its adherents called the "culture wars."

As a grass-roots movement, the Religious Right generally reflected local concerns during the early 1970s. Efforts such as purging the local library of works that the Religious Right deemed morally questionable, along with attempts to ban the teaching of evolution and sex education, dominated the movement's agenda throughout the early 1970s. But even in this early period the Religious Right saw a need to develop a national agenda. By the mid-1970s the Religious Right had taken public stands on issues as diverse as the SALT II Treaty (they were against it), the relinquishment of the Panama Canal (they were against it), and even taxation (they were against it).

In 1976 the election of President Jimmy Carter, an evangelical, was seen as a triumph for the Religious Right, but Carter's reluctance to toe a conservative line quickly led to dissatisfaction among rank-and-file members of the Religious Right. By the late 1970s, more and more members of the Religious Right looked outside their immediate community in search of a politician who would endorse their agenda.

In his personal life Ronald Reagan did not exemplify any of the values the Religious Right claimed to hold dear. Not only was he divorced, but his second wife had been pregnant at the time of their marriage. His political record also offered little that should have appealed to the Religious Right. As governor of California, Reagan had endorsed measures that helped legalize abortion and that sought to prevent discrimination against homosexuals.[12] But Reagan was also an adept politician who quickly recognized the potential power of this very vocal minority group. Adopting the language of the Religious Right, Reagan assiduously courted their vote. Following his election as president in 1980, Reagan rewarded this support by appointing leading figures associated with the Religious Right to high positions within his government.

The nomination of Koop as surgeon general was just one such appointment. Koop had first won credibility with the Religious Right because of his long-standing opposition to abortion, and he was widely considered by the Religious Right to be an outstanding candidate for the position of the nation's First Doctor.[13] But Koop was not the only conservative nominated for a high-ranking position during this period. Within the same twelve-month span in which Reagan nominated Koop, he also appointed Marjory Mecklenburg, the president of American Citizens Concerned for Life, to head the Department of Education's

Federal Office of Adolescent Pregnancy Problems.[14] Mecklenburg's and Koop's nominations were part of a broader pattern of appointments, all of which ensured that federal institutions began to reflect the views of those who opposed both sex education and the sexual revolution of the 1960s.

Pressure from the Right also led the Reagan administration to advocate harsher measures to limit sex education, both directly and indirectly. In 1981 the administration attempted to promulgate "the squeal rule." This rule would have required federally funded clinics to notify the parents of un-emancipated minors who sought contraceptives. While the distinction here seems clear—the regulation was imposed on those who sought contraceptives, not those who sought education on contraceptives—the tendency of teens to seek both educational materials and contraceptives simultaneously was such that the squeal rule, if it had ever been implemented, would have had a chilling effect on the dispersal of educational materials at federally funded clinics.

In advocating policies that sought to limit access to contraceptives, officials in the Reagan administration believed that they were endorsing the views of the majority on "moral" issues. American views on sex, sex education, and the availability of contraceptives were, however, extremely complex. While it is impossible to point to one dominant view on sex and sex education, most Americans sought a middle path. Interviewed as just a "voice from across the nation" in the mid-1980s, Anna Hill called for a sex education program that addressed both the ideal and the reality of sexual behavior. "I would," Hill said, "stress abstinence . . . but if [kids] buckled to peer pressure [and had sex], I'd want them to be protected."[15]

"Evaluating Everything in Terms of Scripture"

In 1976, when the nation's first evangelical president, Jimmy Carter, had been elected, the Religious Right had been elated to have one of their own in the White House. As a Democrat, Carter did not completely share the agenda of this hard-line conservative faction. In fact, much to the dismay of the Religious Right, Carter operated very much as a moderate. However, Carter's evangelical background did lead him to make concessions to the growing power of this new and very vocal faction. Under Carter, for example, funding for global programs on population control was cut in accordance with the wishes of many evangelical and fundamentalist Protestants who condemned both contraception and abortion.[16]

But these small concessions were insufficient to appease the Religious Right. Angered at Carter's refusal to push harder on the many issues that concerned them, the Religious Right united to provide crucial support to Ronald Reagan. Although Reagan would also fail to address the concerns of the Religious Right on issues relating to abortion and contraception, his administration would be characterized by a growing antipathy toward sex education. Along with his many cuts to entitlement programs and other initiatives associated with Johnson's War on Poverty, Reagan also called for deep cuts in family-planning initiatives and programs. Sex education programs, especially those aimed at teenagers and schoolchildren, came in for increasingly harsh scrutiny.

In nominating C. Everett Koop as surgeon general, Reagan believed he had selected someone who shared the views of his most conservative supporters. Like many of Reagan's supporters, Koop was an evangelical Christian, having been born again at the age of thirty-two. Koop was frank about his beliefs, admitting, "I attempted to evaluate everything in terms of Scripture."[17] He even viewed his own practice of medicine from the perspective of his Christianity. In 1974, for example, when he separated conjoined twins, he explained the operation's success to a reporter by saying, "Claiming the righteousness of Jesus Christ, I said 'We're going to win.' And we did." And in 1982, after assuming the position of surgeon general, Koop said, "I knew I was to practice my Christianity through my [medicine]." At the same time that Koop made these statements, however, he also insisted on his ability to differentiate between the physician and the Christian, a rather startling contradiction and one that was in many ways typical of Koop himself.[18]

Koop's insistence on his ability to differentiate between the physician and the Christian would ultimately become the hallmark of his tenure as surgeon general. As Koop became the nation's foremost advocate for better sex education, his ability to make this differentiation would come to shape the Public Health Service's sex education programs. But Koop's desire to straddle two worlds would also bring both the Public Health Service and Koop himself under attack as the AIDS crisis and the already soaring rate of teenage pregnancy escalated.

Why Sex Education?

In 1980, American girls and their counterparts in Europe became sexually active at roughly the same age. But all similarities ended there. American teens were almost twice as likely as their European counterparts to become pregnant.

To public health experts, it was obvious why European governments were so much more successful at lowering pregnancy rates. In Europe, a variety of family-planning programs provided easy access to inexpensive contraceptives. European governments had also developed and implemented comprehensive sex education programs that were committed to preventing pregnancy as opposed to promoting chastity.[19]

Admirable as public health experts found the European model to be, it could not be transported to the United States. Europeans, whether Swedish, Danish, or French, overwhelmingly shared a religion and ethnicity with their fellow countrymen and women. This shared identity meant that their views on sex education tended to be fairly uniform. In America, the situation was radically different. Diverse religious beliefs as well as different racial and ethnic identities have made it all but impossible for the federal government to develop and implement a uniform sex education campaign, one that can be accepted by a majority of Americans. Adding to this problem has been the decentralized nature of the American school system, which prioritizes local control over federal or even state control.

Since the first sex education campaign sponsored by the Public Health Service in 1919, these intertwined issues of local control and diverse populations had caused difficulties for the Public Health Service. The Reagan administration's strong emphasis on state and local control meant that these obstacles had the potential to become insurmountable. That they did not was in many ways to Koop's credit. Early on in the nomination process, Koop had indicated to friends and colleagues his desire to use the position of surgeon general as a bully pulpit.[20] But Koop also sought to ensure that Americans looked to one place—the Public Health Service—for information on any major public health issue.

Koop believed that the Public Health Service needed an iconic image that would raise its visibility. By stepping forward to speak publicly on topics ranging from tobacco to sex education, Koop became the face of public health in America. Before 1981, less than 1 percent of Americans had been able to identify any surgeon general by name or by picture. But within a few years of Koop's appointment, it was almost impossible to open a newspaper or magazine or to turn on the television or radio and not see his face or hear his voice. With his Captain Ahab beard, his insistence on wearing the uniform of the Service, and his eagerness to speak in any available forum, Koop was easily and instantly recognizable.[21] Contributing to Koop's visibility was his willingness to speak on any issue, however controversial. As *Time* put it, Koop "has an opinion which he will give you with great capacity at high speed," and, the article added, he had an opinion on *everything*.[22] While Koop's very vocal opinions were not always welcome, his insistence that his opinions were backed by science had a strong appeal for most Americans. By 1986 a public relations firm had discovered that not only were the overwhelming majority of Americans able to recognize Koop, they also trusted him more than almost any other nationally known figure.[23] And with that trust had come an odd sort of love. When the editors of *USA Weekend* included Koop in a list entitled "Six Sexy Guys and Why We Like

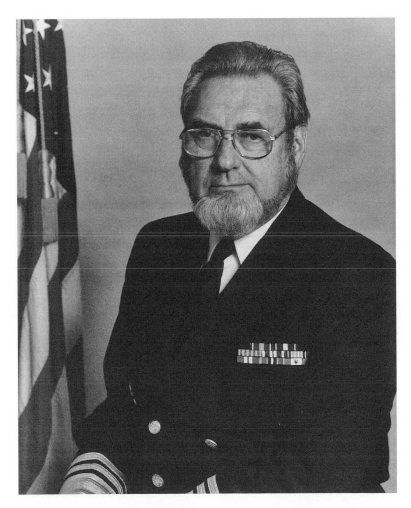

During the 1980s, Surgeon General C. Everett Koop had one of the most trusted faces in government (ca. 1980s). Department of Health and Human Services.

'Em," they gushed that their love stemmed from the fact that "we're partial to a man in uniform." But the sexiness of this elderly uniformed pediatrician notwithstanding, it was Koop's reputation for candor on public health issues that had really precipitated the love.[24]

By the mid-1980s, Koop's fame—and Americans' love of him—had finally led Americans to look to one source for information about the most glaring public health issues of the day. That place was the Public Health Service, or more specifically its surgeon general, C. Everett Koop.

Becoming a Cool Dude

The advent of the AIDS crisis did not completely push concerns about syphilis, gonorrhea, and teenage pregnancy to the sidelines. Throughout the 1980s the Public Health Service continued to advocate for aggressive and comprehensive sex education programs to battle unwanted pregnancies and venereal diseases, or, as they were now coming to be called, sexually transmitted diseases. But while federally funded sex education programs continued to address these traditional problems, it was the AIDS crisis that pushed the Service into developing and implementing the most innovative sex education program ever used in the United States.

The Public Health Service had been astonishingly slow to deal with the AIDS crisis. This tardiness stemmed in part from the structure of federal budgets, which are generally planned one to two years in advance. During the early years of the AIDS crisis federal officials had grossly underestimated the threat AIDS posed and failed to provide comprehensive, extensive, and dedicated funding for AIDS programs. But by 1984, with the Public Health Service coming under vehement attack for failing to address AIDS aggressively, Koop was eager to engage with this issue publicly.

In 1985 Koop finally broke the silence that had been imposed upon him by the Reagan administration by giving his first public interview on AIDS. The interview did not appear in a public health or medical journal. Instead, Koop's comments were published in an evangelical journal, *Christianity Today*. The decision to speak first in *Christianity Today* was a politic move, as it demonstrated to those on the Right that Koop was not prepared to break with his Christianity in order to discuss AIDS. But this approach also had the potential to cause the same problems earlier surgeons general had experienced when dealing with Christian groups such as the YMCA or the Knights of Columbus. Groups that endorsed socially conservative views on sex were unlikely to provide support for those who called for aggressive and comprehensive sex education programs. As Koop would later come to understand, developing the middle road that Anna Hill, that voice of the people interviewed early on in the AIDS crisis, and her fellow Americans wanted would prove to be no easy task.

While Koop's interview in *Christianity Today* may have antagonized many on the Left who deplored his speaking about medical matters in a religious forum, the interview did open the door for him to take a public stance on AIDS and sex education. Shortly after the interview appeared, Koop was asked to prepare a comprehensive report on AIDS. This would be not only Koop's most public statement on AIDS but also the most public statement on AIDS made by the Public Health Service to date.

Describing the writing of the report as "walking a tightrope," Koop followed in the footsteps of his predecessors by reaching out to groups both within and outside the government to prepare the report. The National Education Association, the American Medical Association, the United States Catholic Conference, the Washington Business Group on Health, the National Coalition of Black Lesbians and Gays, and the American Council of Life Insurance all eagerly provided advice. Ultimately, however, the report, issued in October 1986, was written primarily by Koop himself, with input from a dozen close advisors.[25]

The Surgeon General's Report on Acquired Immunity Deficiency Syndrome followed in a long line of surgeon general's reports. The first of these reports had been released in 1964, when Luther Terry had issued *The Report of the Surgeon General on Smoking*. Successive surgeons general had followed Terry's lead, and the previous two decades had seen a series of reports being published by the Public Health Service. The majority of these reports dealt with smoking. By issuing the first in what would become a series of reports on public health issues relating to sex, Koop radically altered the structure of these reports.

Although these reports were ostensibly intended for the general public, both their length and the density of their prose meant that they were rarely read by those outside the public health community. Koop's report on AIDS was quite different. To begin with, it was only thirty-six pages long. In clear, succinct, and jargon-free prose, the report began with a simple description of AIDS and an overview of the "present situation" in the United States with respect to the spread of the disease. A brief explanation of how AIDS was transmitted and a candid discussion of how to protect oneself from it followed, as did a discussion of the future of the disease and its impact on public health. According to the report, AIDS was "no longer the concern of any one segment of society." Paralleling previous sex education documents, which had made similar claims in the fight against venereal disease and unwanted pregnancies, Koop insisted that AIDS "is the concern of us all," and that "information and education" were the nation's "only weapons against AIDS."[26]

Despite its brevity, the report was extremely explicit and detailed. Pictures of condoms were included, and there were frank references to vaginal, anal, and oral intercourse. Equally blunt were discussions of the myths regarding AIDS: "You *cannot* get AIDS from casual social contact . . . such as shaking hands, hugging, social kissing, crying, coughing or sneezing," the report stated firmly. AIDS also cannot be transmitted via "toilets, doorknobs, telephones, office machinery, or household furniture." And for those who wanted more detailed information, the report also explained that "you cannot get AIDS from body massages, masturbation, or any non-sexual contact."[27]

This type of candid approach differed from that endorsed by previous surgeons general. During the 1930s Surgeon General Thomas Parran had believed that encouraging people to be tested for venereal disease was more important than providing accurate information, and to this end he had allowed, and even endorsed, myths about the disease.[28] Now, in 1986, Koop and his fellow advisors rejected such equivocation, in the belief that Americans who had experienced the sexual revolution would be comfortable admitting to sexual encounters that might put them at risk. To some degree these were probably accurate assessments of Americans' slightly more open views about sexuality during the 1980s. However, widespread prejudices against homosexuality, which Koop himself viewed as a sin, meant that some men would be reluctant to admit to the risky practice of anal intercourse.

The report was given a wide release. Several newspapers reprinted it in its entirety. The Parent-Teacher Association requested and distributed over 55,000 copies, and congressional legislators sent it to constituents, at least until they ran out of copies. All of this made for a huge audience, which meant there was a potential to antagonize large groups of people. Well aware of the potential for a backlash, Koop justified his report by arguing that understanding AIDS was a "life or death" issue. But even as he made this statement, he acknowledged that "sex education was a buzzword that would . . . drive many conservatives up the wall."[29] And drive them up the wall it did. Within days of the report's release, Koop discovered that he had alienated a great number of his conservative supporters. Among those who launched early criticisms of Koop were William

Buckley, the conservative writer, Phyllis Schlafly, the founder and president of the conservative Eagle Forum, Robert Novak, the conservative columnist, and Gary Bauer, Reagan's undersecretary of education. To counter some of this criticism, Koop decided to speak directly to the Christian community. He appeared on the Christian Broadcast Network, and he spoke in the large fundamentalist church of which Jerry Falwell was the pastor. Koop clearly saw himself building bridges between science and religious belief. To his credit, Koop actually acknowledged a division that more recent surgeons general had seen but sought to gloss over: the division between the way in which those who prioritized religious belief and those who prioritized science spoke about sex education.

Koop saw this split more clearly than his predecessors had because he himself exemplified it. Previous surgeons general had been predominantly practicing Christians, but they had also been liberal Christians within the context of their culture and society. As an evangelical Christian, Koop knew and often shared the views of those in the Religious Right. But he was also a physician, a scientist, as he so firmly asserted. And this led him to view sex education in a way that was at times diametrically opposed to what he endorsed as an evangelical Christian. Nowhere was this division more evident than in his discussions of homosexuality. For Koop, homosexuality was a sin—a belief that would not endear him to the gay and lesbian community. But he was prepared to temper his views on homosexuality if it enabled him to teach homosexuals and heterosexuals alike the importance of safe sex practices.

The Surgeon General's Report on Acquired Immune Deficiency Syndrome was in many ways an illustration of Koop at his best in straddling the fence. The report acknowledged, without comment, the diversity of opinions about sexuality and homosexuality in America. It stated that "some Americans have difficulties in dealing with the subjects of sex, sexual practices, and alternate lifestyles." "Many Americans," it continued, "are opposed to homosexuality, promiscuity, and prostitution."[30] Although the Reagan administration and many on the Right wished Koop to make a more sweeping statement asserting that "*all* Americans" opposed these behaviors, Koop refused to do so. He believed that this assertion would color and sharply limit his message about the need for sex education.[31] But he also refused to condemn or lecture those who were "opposed to homosexuality" on the need for tolerance, and his references to homosexuality as a sin made it clear where he stood on this issue. For Koop, the issue was complex: "People get AIDS by doing things that most people do not do and do not approve of. So when you [make] . . . a decision about AIDS you must consider" how your words will affect "the way the decision-maker thinks and acts."[32] The key, Koop believed, was to reach the decision maker, the person who was making choices about behaviors that might expose him or her to AIDS. All other concerns were irrelevant in the context of sex education.

Koop also carefully crafted his language to strike a balance. An early version of the report had used street slang to discuss sexual behavior. This was in keeping with a longstanding tradition at the Public Health Service. Pamphlets produced in the early twentieth century right up through the 1970s had often used words such as *whore* or *the clap*. In a radical break with this tradition, Koop made a calculated decision to use scientific language. Unlike his predecessors, especially those in the early twentieth century, Koop was speaking to a population that was highly literate and fairly conversant with basic scientific terms. This gave him options that had been unavailable to his predecessors. But Koop's decision to use scientific terms also took other factors into account. On a very basic level, he was concerned that a discussion of sex using street slang "would turn off a lot of the people [he] wanted to reach."[33] Neutral, scientific language also allowed readers to disassociate themselves from much of the emotional baggage associated with AIDS and sexual behavior, and it underscored that the Public Health Service was a scientific, and therefore knowledgeable and unbiased, entity.

But if the report used nonjudgmental and clinical terms, it was also extraordinarily explicit. It made references not to *body fluids* but rather to *semen* and to *vaginal secretions*. These terms went a long way to removing ambiguity from the minds of most readers.

The release of the report was accompanied by a series of television ads. Koop also did what he did best: he took every opportunity offered to speak publicly about the report and its implications. Sex education, Koop now insisted, needed to begin at a very young age, preferably kindergarten. Sex education should stress abstinence and monogamy, but it should also include frank discussions about how condoms could provide protection against AIDS. Koop's approach to sex education differed dramatically from that advocated by his fellow officials in the Reagan administration. Secretary of Education William Bennett strongly condemned this approach, noting that while sex education that included a discussion of condoms might be "clinically correct, it was morally bankrupt."[34]

In many ways *The Surgeon General's Report on Acquired Immune Deficiency Syndrome* and the media blitz that accompanied it were a success. Despite criticism from the Religious Right, the media and most Americans hailed the report as "no-nonsense."[35] Jeff Levi, executive director of the National Gay and Lesbian Task Force, noted that the report "dramatically altered the level of public discussion on AIDS [by shifting it] from moral judgment to public health."[36] Richard Dunne, executive director of New York's Gay Men's Health Crisis, the oldest and largest AIDS service organization, agreed: "The report was even better than I could have imagined."[37] The editor of the *Atlanta Journal Constitution* wrote that Koop's background as a conservative evangelical combined with his no-nonsense approach to sex education might enable him "to make some headway with those who don't yet understand the dangers of our national reluctance to teach our children about sex."[38] Even Koop's former adversaries such as Congressmen Henry Waxman and Ted Kennedy stepped forward with praise. This praise may have taken some of the sting out of the criticism Koop had received from Phyllis Schlafly, Gary Bauer, and a host of others on the Right, but in a twist that demonstrates the complexity of his character, Koop claimed that his religious belief, not the support of his former opponents, provided him with the greatest comfort during the period in which he came under attack.

The AIDS report actually led Koop into areas in which he himself was deeply uncomfortable. As a public health expert he advocated a more public discussion of sex, sexuality, and sexually transmitted diseases. But as an evangelical Christian he was "deeply saddened by what had happened to America's sexual morality."[39]

Koop's sorrow at what he viewed as a decline in America's sexual standards remained a key concern for him. But his own conflicted views on sex education had a strong appeal to Americans. In 1988 Koop gave a series of interviews and public talks and wrote several articles on AIDS. When he spoke to a Christian audience in 1988, Koop was up-front about the need for Americans to protect themselves through the use of condoms. He also discussed and prioritized abstinence. For this audience, many of whom viewed Koop as one of their own, the message was clear: abstinence was central to the fight against AIDS or any other public health problem associated with sex. Just a few months earlier Koop had spoken to a very different audience at Cardozo High School in Washington, D.C. Here too Koop stressed abstinence, but he also discussed condoms. For this audience, composed predominantly of students, public health experts, and Washington's more liberal politicians, Koop's message was loud and clear: "If you're a man," Koop thundered, "you should wear a condom from start to finish. If you're a woman, you should make sure that your partner wears a condom from start to finish." For those who still had doubts, "the proper use of a condom is a person's best defense against the passing of the AIDS virus during sexual intercourse."[40] In keeping with his views on AIDS and condoms, Koop's speech also provided information intended to assist drug users who were at risk of contracting the AIDS virus through a dirty needle. By the time Koop had wrapped up his talk, the students were deeply impressed by his frankness. "You tell that general he's a cool dude for coming down here," one admiring student told a reporter.[41]

Given Koop's strong Christianity and the ways in which his religious beliefs shaped his views of sexuality, the vision of Koop as a "cool dude" was not necessarily accurate. But when the majority of Americans assessed what Koop was saying, where he was saying it, and why he was saying it, they did so through the filter of their own prejudices. It was no surprise, then, that Americans who heard Koop speak, in their schools, churches, and community centers, often took away from these encounters a belief that Koop shared their values.

Not all audiences embraced Koop, of course. For many in the Religious Right, Koop's nuanced message, which stressed abstinence, monogamy, and the use of condoms, was completely unacceptable. But in attacking Koop, many of his critics focused only on those parts of Koop's message with which they disagreed. Nicknaming Koop "the condom king," they insisted that the government's sex education message should stress abstinence only. Discussions of abstinence could never be coupled with discussions of condoms. Koop clearly felt blindsided by the attacks from those whom he considered fellow Christians, yet these attacks could have been foreseen. Like his critics, Koop had a history of taking an all-or-nothing approach on different public health issues. Just as his critics rejected a nuanced view of sex education, so too had Koop rejected a nuanced view of abortion during the 1970s. But the vitriol heaped on Koop during this period also stemmed from the fact that during the 1970s he had been seen as being on the side of the Religious Right. For those who had entertained high hopes that Koop would lead their charge, his refusal to take their side on the issue of sex education seemed a bitter betrayal.

By the mid-1980s Koop had become the public health expert and advocate he had claimed to be in 1981. He had also mastered the high-wire act that most Beltway politicians only dream of attaining. While he did not accomplish the impossible—reaching those on the extremes of either side of the political divide—Koop routinely struck a chord with audiences who endorsed mainstream views on both the Left and the Right. How calculated his tactics were in achieving this success is not clear. What is clear is that Koop was driven by what he saw as his primary goal: the prevention of a fatal disease through any and all means possible. Whether these steps toward preventing the spread of AIDS entailed using a condom or practicing abstinence was of no real concern to Surgeon General C. Everett Koop and, by extension, the federal government.

"It's What You Do"

In 1988, as international experts on AIDS gathered in London, the *Boston Globe* remarked that American officials "should be shamefaced." Experts in forty other countries had developed comprehensive materials designed to educate their citizens about AIDS. In the United States, however, only *The Surgeon General's Report on Acquired Immunity Deficiency Syndrome* had addressed the growing crisis with candor and in detail. Of special concern to the *Globe*'s editors—and, they claimed, to all Americans—was the new AIDS brochure that had recently been developed by Otis Bowen, secretary of the Department of Health and Human Services, the newly configured department in which the Public Health Service now resided.

Unlike Koop's *Report*, Bowen's "inane" pamphlet, the *Globe* complained, has "only a minimal reference to condoms and an aside about gay men not being the only ones who can get AIDS." True, the slogan "America Responds to AIDS" could be found on every page, but the brochure provided no real information on how Americans could or should respond to the threat. Instead, it simply urged Americans to "say no to sex." But this was not the only problem with the pamphlet. In a complaint reminiscent of the old joke in which the diner complains that the food is terrible and served in tiny portions, the *Globe* pointed out that the limited print run of the pamphlet and the Public Health Service's traditional approach of simply distributing it to local health departments, YMCAs, and selected companies and organizations meant that few Americans would even read the pamphlet. Something more was needed. Perhaps, the *Globe*'s editors suggested, an educational pamphlet about AIDS should be sent to every American household.[42]

Responding to these and other calls, in 1988 Congress, public health experts, and federal officials decided to take the dramatic step of directly providing all Americans with information about AIDS. This step would actually force the Public Health Service to write and endorse a uniform pamphlet about AIDS. Not only would the government's message have to be uniform (which could provoke great animosity from groups on either end of the political spectrum),

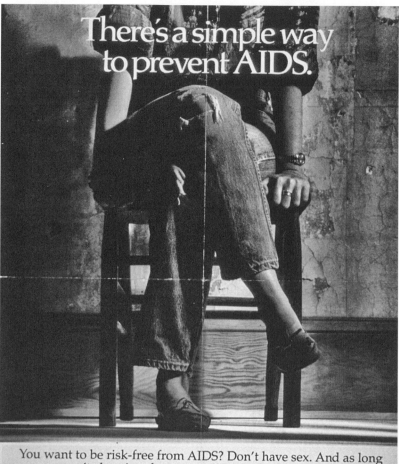

There's a simple way to prevent AIDS.

You want to be risk-free from AIDS? Don't have sex. And as long as you aren't shooting drugs, you'll be fine. No worries about who's slept around, who's had blood tests, and whether your condoms are latex or not. 1-800-342-AIDS. For the hearing impaired, 1-800-AIDS-TTY.

AMERICA RESPONDS TO AIDS

Posters also reinforced the message that abstinence was the proper response to the AIDS crisis (ca. 1980s). Department of Health and Human Services.

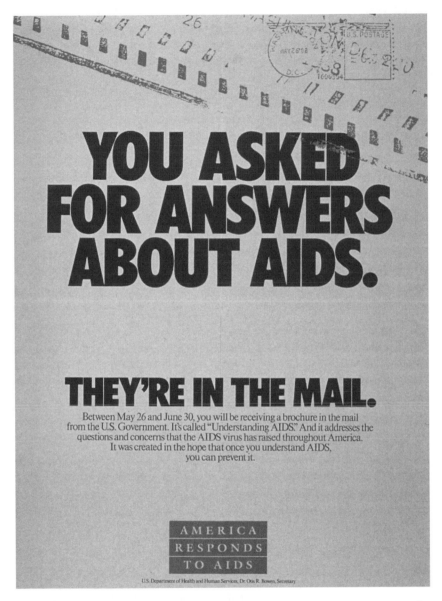

The AIDS mailer was widely advertised even before it was released (1988). Department of Health and Human Services.

it would also have to be concise and clear. Koop's actions of the previous two years had laid substantial groundwork for this new pamphlet. The PHS now had a baseline report (*The Surgeon General's Report*) on which to draw to create a short and very simple brochure. Koop's reputation as one of the most trusted men in America, if not the sexiest, also ensured that any public health message that he backed would have a wide appeal.

Congress appropriated $20 million for the mailing of the brochure, and wary of the potential for political battles, legislators insisted that the mailer be cleared by health officers, not White House officials. Preparing the mailer became a logistical nightmare. Copies were prepared in several Spanish dialects and even Braille. Presses ran for twenty-four hours a day for six weeks, consuming 20,900 miles of paper. Nearly two hundred trucks were deployed to carry the 114 million copies of the brochure, and the Public Health Service wound up using railroad cars to store the mailer before its release. By early May of 1988 the AIDS brochure was ready for what would be the largest mass mailing in American history.[43]

The mailer consisted of just seven pages, and the text itself was interspersed with various images. Lynn Herring, the official at CDC who oversaw the mailing, described the pamphlet by saying, "It's not who you are, *it's what you do*."[44] This message was in direct opposition to the views endorsed by William Bennett, Reagan's secretary of education. Bennett and his supporters in the administration believed that discussions of AIDS should begin with a discussion of morality and the ways in which morality should shape sexual behavior. In other words, Bennett believed that AIDS *was* about who you are.[45]

The mailer provided information about "what you can do to stop AIDS." On a basic level, it sought to provide the "best information available" on AIDS. More narrowly, the mailer also sought to educate Americans both on how to protect themselves and on how to treat fellow citizens who were suffering from AIDS. The mailer attempted to eradicate prevalent myths about AIDS. Predominant among these was the belief that AIDS was confined to the homosexual population. "In spite of what you may have heard, the number of heterosexual[s with AIDS] is growing," the mailer stated. It also countered a number of common misconceptions: "You won't get the AIDS virus through everyday contact . . . you won't get AIDS from a mosquito bite . . . you won't get AIDS from saliva, sweat, tears, urine, or a bowel movement . . . [and] you won't get AIDS from a kiss."[46]

The mailer was sent in a sealed packet, and Americans were cautioned before opening the packet that "some of the issues involved in this brochure may not be things you are used to discussing openly." Like *The Surgeon General's Report on Acquired Immune Deficiency Syndrome*, the mailer used detailed and highly clinical language. But unlike the *Report*, which had been made available only to those who requested it, the AIDS mailer, with its frank references to "semen and vaginal fluids" and "oral, anal, and vaginal intercourse," arrived in the mailboxes of *all* Americans, whether they had requested the information or not.

Public reaction to the mailer was immediate. A surprising 82 percent of Americans read all or part of it. Call centers that had been set up to deal with any questions people might have after reading the pamphlet were flooded with calls. In Minneapolis the science reporter for the city's largest paper noted that the mailer was "just good, lifesaving reading." It did "an excellent job of simplifying the complex" issue of safe and unsafe practices while "presenting information in an easy-to-read form." Best of all, it avoided being judgmental.[47] In Boston, editors at the *Globe* cried, "Hooray for the United States Congress for insisting that the government get a plain-speaking pamphlet on AIDS out to the public."[48] But, as the *Chicago Tribune* pointed out, the effectiveness of the message was still in doubt. After all, "just as some people still smoke and ignore seat belts, some will disregard warnings about AIDS."[49]

More worrisome, however, was the fact that the AIDS mailer gave ammunition to a growing and very vocal group who opposed sex education programs and materials that mentioned condoms. "Disinformation abounds," said an enraged Judie Brown, the president of the American Life League. The brochure, she charged, "caters to such lifestyles as homosexuality and bisexuality by avoiding even a modest encouragement toward a type of sexual relationship designed by nature for man and woman to become one in marriage."[50] Jerry Falwell, whom Koop had spent time courting, grumbled that the simple message "no sex outside of marriage would have saved taxpayers' money."[51] Abstinence, stressed opponents of sex education, was the only suitable message for sex education materials, especially those funded with taxpayer money.

The AIDS mailer actually did advocate abstinence. But it also advocated the use of condoms for those who were unprepared to practice abstinence. Ironically, where Koop had won tremendous support from many Americans because they saw him through the filter of their own prejudices and beliefs, he was heavily criticized by those in the Religious Right who read the mailer through the filter of their own biases. Reading the criticisms of those who attacked the mailer, one might conclude that the Public Health Service had omitted any mention of abstinence. Yet the Public Health Service openly acknowledged that abstinence was the best protection against AIDS, and Koop himself continued to be a strong advocate for abstinence. But for those who believed that all discussions of sexual behavior should be morally based, any deviation from the set message of abstinence—or, more simply, any shading of the issue to include those whose actions did not conform to the standards of the Religious Right—was simply unacceptable.

If the mailer, which was aimed at the middle, had antagonized those on the Far Right who believed that it went too far, why did it not antagonize those on the Far Left who might claim that it had not gone far enough? In many ways the mailer benefited from both the Public Health Service's failure to address the crisis early on and its strong association with Koop. The contentious hearings that had marked his confirmation had made many on the Left fear that Koop would be unable to separate his religious beliefs from his work as surgeon general. Expectations were so low that any reasonable action Koop took to address the spread of AIDS would be seen as a surprise and a measure of his growth in office. But Koop also benefited from having already taken highly public and highly controversial stances on issues as wide-ranging as cigarette smoking and the rights of handicapped children. Unlike previous surgeons general, Koop had made himself extraordinarily visible long before he stepped forward to speak on sex education. By 1988 most Americans viewed Koop as a man who was prepared to champion any difficult or unpopular view, provided that the science was on his side. Perhaps more important, the repeated attacks Koop had endured from those on the Right gave him political credibility with many on the Left. As a result, when the PHS released the AIDS mailer, even those on the Far Left were prepared to endorse and support it because it was directly associated with Koop. Rightly or wrongly, these Americans saw Koop, and by extension the Public Health Service, as being on the Left when it came to sex education.

While the AIDS mailer resulted in strong reactions from those on the Left who hailed Koop as a hero and those on the Right who viewed him as a traitor, its impact on its intended audience—average Americans—was more difficult to assess. Follow-up studies by the Public Health Service indicated that the mailer answered some of the more basic questions Americans had about AIDS and its transmission (although the persistence of myths regarding AIDS would seem to indicate that the mailer did not have as sweeping an impact as its creators would have liked).[52] But despite being accompanied by television ads, the mailer was in many ways a one-shot deal, and sex education, as the PHS has long known, is most effective when its message is constantly repeated in a variety of different formats.

Fall from Grace

Koop's prominence as the most visible symbol of AIDS education made him an easy target for his opponents. In 1989 Koop's already strained relationship with the most conservative members of the Republican party fell apart. The election of George H. W. Bush in 1988 meant that Ronald Reagan, the man who had appointed Koop to office, was no longer able to provide him with support. While Reagan's support for Koop had decreased dramatically as Koop became more and more aggressive about advocating sex education, Koop's former colleagues have noted that the two were similar in temperament. These similarities enabled the two men to get along, even at the height of their disagreements over sex education. Bush and Koop, however, were radically different, and it is unlikely that they would have gotten along, even if Bush had been prepared to endorse Koop's views on sex education.

In 1989 Koop formally resigned from his position as surgeon general. If he felt any bitterness about being forced out by the Bush administration, the eulogies published in the wake of his resignation, both in America and abroad, may have provided some solace.

For Koop, as for many Americans, the issue of sex education was not a political one. Pointing out that he "walk[ed] a fine line [between] being a public health officer and presenting all the things that have to be said about AIDS," Koop insisted that he had "never wanted to politicize the issue of AIDS." Instead, he maintained, his approach had been simply to view the office of the surgeon general as a forum for speaking about public health and medical science. It was, Koop said, others in the Reagan administration and in American society at large who had sought to politicize the issue of AIDS and the publications that he had released in his position as surgeon general.

CHAPTER EIGHT

ABSTINENCE MAKES THE HEART GROW FONDER 1989–2008

Masturbation is a part of sex education and should perhaps be taught.

SURGEON GENERAL JOYCELYN ELDERS (ATTRIBUTED), 1994

Let's face it, sex makes people crazy.

WARD CATES, DIRECTOR OF THE SEXUALLY TRANSMITTED DISEASE PROGRAM, CENTERS FOR DISEASE CONTROL, 1990

T he blogosphere went wild. John McCain's choice of Sarah Palin, a religious conservative and the relatively unknown governor of Alaska, as his vice-presidential nominee sparked almost nonstop rumors as pundits and the general public assessed McCain's choice across the worldwide web. Among the many rumors swirling both in the tabloids and on the Internet were whispers about Palin's oldest daughter. In an attempt to quash the rumors, the Palin family issued a formal statement: "Our beautiful daughter Bristol came to us with news that as parents we knew would make her grow up faster than we had ever planned." Bristol's pregnancy was, Palin's supporters argued, "evidence that they are a normal American family with all the joys and problems." A Republican delegate explained to the *New York Times* that Palin's situation had "every single person . . . thinking 'Oh my gosh, that has happened to me or to someone I know or I am afraid it will.' "[1]

In many ways this delegate was correct. Even as Bristol Palin's pregnancy sparked a major debate in the press and on the Internet about the merits and drawbacks of abstinence-only sex education, pundits found echoes of recent and similar stories of high-profile teens who had also become pregnant. Just nine months before the story about Palin broke, the 2007 Christmas season had wound to a close with the announcement that one of America's cherished teen idols was pregnant. In Concord, Massachusetts, teenagers had gathered around the cafeteria lunch tables to discuss Jamie Lynn Spears' surprise announcement. "There's no excuse for not using contraceptives," one student grumbled. Her classmates agreed. It was, they all pointed out, "unrealistic to think that sixteen-year-olds would not have sex." Someone, they insisted, "should have talked to Ms. Spears about contraception."[2] But who? Nine years before Spears' pregnancy made the news, a small federally funded organization in Louisiana had cheerfully stated that "December was an excellent month" for preaching abstinence as "we were able to focus on the virgin birth and make it apparent that God desire[s] sexual purity as a way of life."[3] A year before Spears' pregnancy, a similar media frenzy had developed around the pregnancy of another sixteen-year-old actress. Keisha Castle-Hughes had not only become pregnant as an unwed teenager, she was also slated to play the Virgin Mary in an upcoming film, *The Nativity*. The pope and many on the Right expressed indirect and direct disapproval.[4]

The very public struggles of these teenage girls led to heated debates across the Internet and in the media. The press was for the most part sharply divided over whether these teenage pregnancies presented an opportunity to teach abstinence or the importance of using birth control. Many of the more famous pundits, whose fortunes rested on their close association with either the Left or the Right, chose the simple route. For Bill O'Reilly on the Right, this meant condemning Hollywood and those associated with it (Jamie Lynn Spears and Keisha Castle-Hughes) while providing support for the Palins.[5] For Bill Maher on the Left, it meant establishing a website designed to "free Levi," the boyfriend of Bristol Palin. But more thoughtful pundits and columnists used these events to force a conversation about abstinence-only education, its effectiveness, and the need to speak candidly to teens about contraception.

Pundits charged that no one had spoken to Spears, Palin, or Castle-Hughes about contraception, a charge that was not particularly surprising. During the 1980s the Public Health Service had mounted a successful sex education program that included candid discussions about the use of contraceptives to prevent both unwanted pregnancies and the spread of sexually transmitted diseases. In the short term the PHS had won the battle for a comprehensive sex education campaign. But after the election of President George H. W. Bush in 1988, it became clear that the Public Health Service had lost the war. During the two decades that followed the presidency of the first President Bush, comprehensive sex education programs did not completely disappear, but they declined in number across America. In their place, schools and a variety of other organizations implemented programs advocating abstinence only.

Rooted in Abstinence

In the 1950s, Prescott Bush, the father of George H. W. Bush, lost a Senate seat when his support of Planned Parenthood became public knowledge. Early in his career the younger Bush had followed in his father's footsteps by supporting and advocating the dissemination of information about birth control. George H. W. Bush had even been an avid supporter of Title X, which had ensured the distribution of contraceptives at federally funded clinics. But by the 1980s, George H. W. Bush found himself in a bind. The mood of the country had shifted to the right, and a growing and very vocal movement condemning both birth control and comprehensive sex education had emerged. Because the proponents of this movement constituted a substantial voting bloc, winning the presidency now required gaining the support of this group.[6] In the 1980s, Bush publicly repudiated his former views on sex education and birth control.

In 1989, when President George H. W. Bush was looking for a new surgeon general, his primary goal was to find one who would please his new constituents on the Far Right. Learning from his predecessor's mistake, Bush was eager to ensure that his nomination was the opposite of the very outspoken and completely uncontrollable former surgeon general C. Everett Koop.

Like Koop, Antonia Novello, a career officer in the Public Health Service, was a pediatrician. But the similarities between the two physicians ended there. As a relatively young officer in the middle of her career, the soft-spoken Novello was characterized in the media and by her peers at the National Institutes of Health (NIH) as "a good soldier who doesn't squawk."[7] Novello did not consistently toe the conservative line on issues relating to sex education, but her tenure did usher in a new age in which the Public Health Service ceased to "squawk" loudly about the necessity of comprehensive sex education.

The government's shift to the right and the implications for federally funded efforts to promote sex education became evident within the first year of Novello's tenure. In 1990, just one year after her appointment, a major survey on Americans' sexual behavior that Congress had wanted was derailed. As the most detailed study of American sexual habits since Alfred Kinsey's work in the 1940s and 1950s, the survey would have determined which Americans were most at risk of contracting a sexually transmitted disease or becoming pregnant unintentionally. Using this information, public health experts could create a sex education program that directly targeted those who were most in need of it. Selling the survey to the American people, however, proved to be trickier than its proponents had imagined. When news of the survey became public, religious and conservative broadcasters took to the airwaves charging that the survey was both an intrusion into the private lives of Americans and an invitation to a more permissive society. In the wake of this barrage of publicity, callers besieged radio and television stations protesting the study. Representative William Dannemeyer, a conservative from Orange County, California, typified the opposition. A sex survey, Dannemeyer complained, would "sway public opinion to liberalize laws regarding homosexuality, pedophilia, anal and oral sex, sex education and teenage pregnancies." In response to this outcry, Congress tabled the survey.[8]

However, the most significant change in the structure of federally funded sex education came in the form of decreased funding for comprehensive sex education—that is, sex education that included discussions of both abstinence and contraceptives. In 1988, over 80 percent of Americans believed that schools should teach sex education, and over 93 percent of American schools provided this type of education. While the actual amount of time most schools spent on such education was limited to a few hours per year, the overwhelming majority of these programs were comprehensive in that they provided information on the ways in which abstinence, monogamy, and contraceptives could prevent sexually transmitted diseases and unwanted pregnancies.[9] But during the presidency of Ronald Reagan, funding for abstinence-only programs began to rise. In 1981, two conservative congressmen, Orrin Hatch of Utah and Jeremiah Denton of Alabama, co-sponsored the Adolescent Family Life Act (AFLA). Included in the Omnibus Budget Reconciliation Act of 1981, the bill had no hearings, and there were no discussions regarding its provisions before it became law. For its supporters, the Act, which promoted chastity, was viewed as a much-needed counterbalance to Title X, which had allowed for contraceptives to be disseminated from clinics receiving federal funds. More important, AFLA channeled funding away from organizations such as Planned Parenthood that provided a broad array of reproductive services, including abortion. Because religious organizations had been at the forefront of the abstinence-only movement, these institutions wound up receiving a substantial amount of the funding provided by AFLA.

The federal government and the Public Health Service had a long history of providing funding for sex education to organizations having religious ties.

Keeping Fit, the Public Health Service's first sex education campaign, had been a collaborative effort with the YMCA. At the time, the YMCA was an overtly religious institution with strong ties to the evangelical Protestant community. J. A. Van Dis, the YMCA official who created the federal program, had even spoken of his desire to have organizations "Christianize" its message, and the PHS had also encouraged churches and other religious institutions to promote discussions of syphilis and gonorrhea among their congregants during this period. However, the PHS never knowingly provided funds to religious institutions to "Christianize" its program, and there is no evidence that federal employees knew of Van Dis' intentions or endorsed his views. More important, there is no evidence that religious organizations used religious symbols or doctrine to promote the government's sex education campaign. But the PHS had come dangerously close to blurring the line between church and state with this early-twentieth-century campaign. By the 1970s, the PHS and the Department of Health, Education, and Welfare had become much more savvy and much more concerned about the potential conflicts that could ensue as a result of this approach. When the PHS and HEW reached out to YMCAs to promote their sex education campaign during this later period, they did so knowing that the YMCA had become a highly secularized institution that did not promote overtly Christian messages, that was not affiliated with any one religious organization, and that welcomed and did not seek to convert non-Christians.

Beginning in the late 1980s, federal officials who administered AFLA became less careful about supervising the government's interactions with religious institutions. AFLA funds went to organizations such as the Catholic facility St. Margaret's Hospital, in Dorchester, Massachusetts. Using federal funds and with the knowledge of federal officials, St. Margaret's created an abstinence-only program that featured materials on "The Church's Teachings on Abortion" and "The Church's Teachings on Artificial Contraception." In 1983 the American Civil Liberties Union (ACLU) sued the federal government, claiming that AFLA, as it was being administered, violated the separation of church and state. The investigation and appeal process took several years, during which attorneys found widespread constitutional violations by the Reagan and Bush administrations. In 1993 the case was finally settled when the Department of Health and Human Services, which administered the program, agreed to provide stricter monitoring of grantees and their programs to ensure that the line between church and state was maintained.[10]

Despite these challenges, AFLA significantly changed the structure of federally funded sex education programs. Between 1988 and 1999, the proportion of teachers who taught in abstinence-only programs rose from 1 in 50 to 1 in 4. Turning away from Surgeon General C. Everett Koop's call to provide comprehensive sex education at the earliest age possible, American schools ceased to provide their students with information on condoms or birth control as a method of preventing sexually transmitted diseases or unwanted pregnancies.[11]

In the absence of comprehensive sex education programs, a surgeon general who prioritized sex education could, as Parran and Koop had demonstrated, make a crucial difference. But although Antonia Novello had worked on issues relating to pediatric AIDS and although she had made children her priority long before she became surgeon general, she was reluctant to use her position to badger an unwilling Bush administration or those on the Right into a reassessment of their growing rejection of comprehensive sex education. In 1992, when Novello released *Parents Speak out for America's Children: Report of the Surgeon General's Conference*, the report contained no references to sex education.

AIDS, however, was an elephant that could not be overlooked, and by the early 1990s Novello was eager to release a surgeon general's report on AIDS that would both serve as a followup to Koop's report and provide information on risk factors that had been unknown in 1986. But here Novello encountered problems. In the spring of 1992 a frustrated Frederick Kroger, head of the AIDS education program at the CDC (the Centers for Disease Control and Prevention), told a congressional subcommittee that the report "was being held until after the election." The report had been lying "fallow since September, 1991" because of fears that its frank language and detailed information would offend Bush's most conservative constituents. While Novello denied that she had allowed the report to be held back for political reasons, the timing of the report's release—which was slated for late 1992 *after* the election—remained suspicious. The delayed release date was even more suspicious as early test marketing of the report in six cities had indicated that a surprising 99 percent of survey respondents thought well of the report and wanted relatives and friends to read it.[12]

In the post-Koop era, there was little in Novello's report that could shock Americans. In fact, Novello's approach to sex education was extremely cautious. Insisting that "families nurture children, provide a supportive environment and teach values and discipline," the report stressed that sex education should begin in the home. Schools were a part of the process, but "the most effective sex education programs support and reinforce the AIDS prevention message given at home."[13] In many ways this emphasis on sex education being taught in the home was a clear response to the concerns of the Religious Right, which had always held that sex education should be provided in the home, not in the schools. This approach had a strong appeal even among those who did not consider themselves part of the Religious Right. After all, who could argue with the idea that individual parents should be allowed to shape the sex education their children received? Unfortunately, studies dating back to the 1920s had demonstrated, over and over again, that many American parents failed to provide their children with any sex education in the home. But even when parents were prepared, in the words of an early-twentieth-century Public Health Service pamphlet, to "do their part" and teach sex education at home, the nature and scope of this education varied widely. If a child learned only abstinence at home, should a school program reinforce that message? But if so, then what kind of program could that school provide to the child who received more comprehensive sex education at home?

Although Novello sidestepped the complicated issues raised by Americans' diverse views on sex and religion, her report did discuss, as her predecessor's had, practical ways in which AIDS could be prevented. Abstinence and monogamy were touted as the best ways to avoid the disease, but readers were also told "if you are not in a [committed and monogamous] . . . relationship and [you] engage in sex you should use a latex condom every time you have sex." Detailed instructions as to how one could and should use condoms followed. These instructions also put to rest persistent rumors regarding the reported failures of condoms: "Condom failure is usually due to a person not using the condom correctly, rather than flaws in the condom itself."[14]

The report did not stand alone. Posters, television ads, and pamphlets describing how Americans could protect themselves from sexually transmitted diseases and unwanted pregnancies were also released during Novello's tenure. But unlike Koop's report, Novello's provoked little to no discussion in the mainstream press of sex, sexually transmitted disease, teenage pregnancy, or sex education. To be fair, Koop's status as a major media figure meant that almost anything Novello did would be seen as anticlimactic. Yet Novello's failures were not limited simply to her inability to develop more innovative ways to provide Americans with sex education. Unlike Koop, she never became the face of the Public Health Service, and unlike Koop, she did not call for widespread dispersal of the government's sex education materials. This failure to agitate for comprehensive sex education or, more simply, to develop more innovative ways to reach Americans, was an indication of trouble ahead.

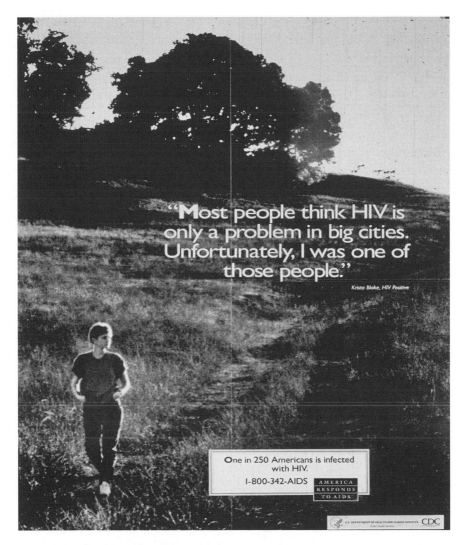

Reminding Americans that sexually transmitted diseases were not confined to urban areas had always been central to the government's sex education campaigns (ca. 1990s). Department of Health and Human Services.

Novello's reluctance to antagonize opponents of comprehensive sex education was shared by her boss, George H. W. Bush. Bush's history as a supporter of Planned Parenthood, Title X, and even *Roe v. Wade* made it unlikely that he could win the Religious Right's complete trust, but he was prepared to try. During his four years as president, Bush used a variety of tactics to push the federal government into endorsing the Religious Right's views on sex education. Among these tactics was the midlevel political appointment. Because most midlevel appointments did not require confirmation from Congress, none of these appointees were required to state publicly their views on sex education. Throughout the Bush presidency, stealth appointments of this type were used to place advocates of abstinence-only programs in crucial positions. Few Americans knew, for example, that Bush had appointed William R. Archer III, a strong opponent of birth control and premarital sex, as the assistant secretary for population affairs in the Department of Health and Human Services. In the grand scheme of things Archer was, as one reporter put it, "a small potato." But this small potato also proved to be a very hot potato. Archer advised the secretary of the Department of Health and Human Services, Louis Sullivan, on contraception, teen sexuality and teen pregnancies, and family-planning services in general. More important, Archer, who advocated abstinence in both his private and public life, was responsible for allocating funds under Title X and the Adolescent Family Life Act.[15]

In the long run, even appointments such as these failed to convince the Religious Right that Bush was on their side. But even as the Religious Right withdrew their support, Bush had dramatically changed the structure of sex education in the United States. Although the settlement of the lawsuit sparked by the Adolescent Family Life Act forced the government to provide greater scrutiny to sex education grants given under the Act, the government had started down a path that prioritized abstinence over comprehensive sex education. There would be, at least over the next fifteen years, no turning back.

"The Wake-up Call"

In 1992, however, many proponents and opponents of comprehensive sex education believed that the election of Bill Clinton would cause a shift in the government's approach to sex education. If nothing else, Clinton's record seemed to indicate that he would emphasize this issue. As governor of Arkansas, Clinton had demonstrated a passionate interest in the broad issue of educational reform. With his wife, Hillary Rodham, he had worked to transform Arkansas' notoriously poor educational system. During the presidential campaign he had also promised to address the growing crisis in health care, the politically tricky issue of gay rights, and growing challenges to legal abortion, all issues that would have a direct impact on the government's approach to sex education. By the time voters on both the Left and the Right entered the voting booth in November 1992, most of them knew that in Clinton they would have a president whose views on sex, sexually transmitted diseases, teenage pregnancy, and sex education differed from those of his predecessor.

If there was any doubt on this issue, voters had only to look at the woman Clinton had appointed as the director of the Arkansas Department of Health. An outspoken African-American pediatrician, Joycelyn Elders had overseen a controversial program to distribute condoms in the state's schools. Throughout the late 1980s and early 1990s, as the number of adolescents who contracted not only syphilis and gonorrhea but also HIV/AIDS rose, school districts from rural Maryland to suburban California had attempted to develop programs to distribute condoms to students. But these distribution programs met with extremely vocal opposition from some parents and community leaders. "This gives a stamp of approval to something we feel is unhealthy and immoral," argued the ultra-conservative Lubavitcher rabbi Abraham Hecht. Proponents of distribution programs countered that "to call abstinence a fantasy is to stretch even the idea of a fantasy." Pointing out that half of the nation's sixteen-year-olds were sexually active, Debra Haffner, the director of the Sexuality Information and Education Council of the United States (SIECUS), insisted that the distribution of condoms was not an immoral act. The immorality, she said, was in those who "say 'just say no or die.'" In calling for condom distribution, Debra Haffner, the director of SIECUS, was breaking with the tradition of her own organization. In its early years SIECUS had advocated abstinence.

Arguments regarding condom use and adolescents were even more complex than many of these simple discussions would seem to indicate. Proponents and opponents of providing adolescents with more and better knowledge as well as contraceptives pointed out the complexity of the issue. Teens "approach sex in neither a logical nor a rational way," Stan Weed, a supporter of abstinence programs from the Institute for Research and Evaluation, pointed out. On the opposite end of the spectrum, Richard P. Keeling, the chair of the American College Health Association's Task Force on AIDS, admitted that the mixed messages teens received with regard to sex simply caused many of them to act in ways contrary to the advice they were receiving in their sex education programs. Congress' failure to sanction the survey on American sexual behavior simply added to the problems, as researchers and educators were forced to guess at most Americans' sexual behavior. While Americans were uncertain about the distribution of condoms in schools during the 1990s, their views shifted over the next few years. By 2007 a report by the Kaiser Family Foundation indicated that 67 percent of Americans favored the distribution of condoms in schools.[16]

In Arkansas, Elders' plan to distribute condoms had backfired not because of opposition from opponents of comprehensive sex education but rather because the condoms distributed to one group of high school students came from a batch with a high percentage of defects. The condoms were recalled, and later studies of the worst batches demonstrated that 95 percent of the condoms were safe, with only 5 percent deemed defective. "Citing her fear that a young person would not bother using a condom at all if he or she knew that it might be defective," Elders opted not to make public the information that the condoms were defective. In Arkansas, the decisions both to release the condoms and to avoid a public announcement of the recall met with harsh criticism. Elders' defense—that she had followed the cardinal rule of public health by acting in the interests of the greatest number of Arkansans by avoiding discussions of the flawed condoms—was overwhelmingly condemned by her opponents.[17]

Elders had no love for the Religious Right, and she had refused to cater to their interests. But she had taken this a step further by repeatedly and very publicly denouncing those on the Far Right throughout her career as director of the Arkansas Department of Health. Statements such as her widely reported comment that the advocates of the Religious Right "love little babies, as long as they're in someone else's uterus," won her few supporters, as did her very public dismissal of the Religious Right as "religious non-Christians." She had also clashed with many of her fellow African Americans, criticizing those who equated her efforts to contain teenage pregnancies with genocide or, even more simply, overt discrimination. In an especially blunt and often quoted comment, Elders had compared unmarried teen mothers to slaves.[18]

By the time Clinton nominated her as his surgeon general in the spring of 1993, it was clear that Elders' decision in the condom recall, combined with her record of being extremely blunt, if not impolitic, would make her a contentious nominee. In June and July of 1993, as Elders' nomination came before Congress, critics and supporters on both sides of the aisle emerged. Pat Robertson, the leader of the Christian Coalition, denounced her as a "way-out radical leftist." Phyllis Schlafly, who had labeled Koop the condom king, nicknamed Elders the condom queen. Janet Parshall, special assistant to the president of the conservative organization Concerned Women of America, labeled Elders "morally reprehensible." Taking a cue from Elders' own rhetoric, Parshall's organization also alleged that the nominee "would like to enslave every child in America to her idea of sexuality education." And from her home state of Arkansas, the Reverend Willis Walker compared Elders to "the midwives of Egypt . . . killing the babies of America."

In response to these and similar outcries, Donna Shalala, Clinton's secretary of the Department of Health and Human Services, said, "Those who would portray Dr. Elders as being radical or out of touch with the desires of the American people are distorting her record." Elders, Shalala noted with some irritation, "supports comprehensive health training . . . but that does not mean inappropriate sex education . . . for young children, as her critics suggest." Elders also found support among her fellow Methodists and other mainstream Protestant and Jewish groups. The director of the United Church of Christ's Office for Church in Society summed up the sentiments of many of his fellow liberal Protestants, saying, "We are frankly disturbed to see [Elders'] candidacy used . . . to attack sex education, birth control, people with AIDS and a woman's right to choose abortion." It was Koop all over again, pundits gleefully noted.[19]

But was it really? One of the major obstacles to Koop's nomination had been his lack of experience in the field of public health. Even Elders' most vocal critics could not claim that she lacked experience. Much of her career had been spent in this field. As her hearing dragged on, her experience and expertise were put under the microscope. By September, Elders had won over enough of her critics to gain the nomination, and converts such as Republican Senator Bob Packwood enthusiastically endorsed her, saying that she was "the wake-up call we need to hear." But as Elders headed off to put on the uniform of the surgeon general on September 8, 1993, even her supporters worried that her reputation for outspokenness would be her undoing. Senator Nancy Kassebaum fretted that she was a bit of "a diamond in the rough."[20]

Ultimately Elders' unwillingness to bow to political forces would prove to be her undoing. But while Elders' tenure as surgeon general lasted less than two years, her outspoken calls for improved sex education forced the issue back to the forefront of American politics.

The M Word

As tensions over her nomination mounted, Elders traveled to New York City to receive an award from the Academy for Educational Development. At the award ceremony, she sounded an alarm: "Our children are out in the ocean drowning while we're sitting on the beach worried and talking about whose values and whose morals we are going to teach."[21] For Elders, the fundamental problems facing the nation were the "issues of teenage pregnancy and making every child a planned, wanted child." Echoing her predecessors in the 1960s and 1970s, she insisted that poverty often stemmed from teenage or unwanted pregnancies. The strong and very clear connections among poverty, ignorance, and poor health meant that providing American children with comprehensive sex education and a full understanding of the ways to prevent disease should, Elders said, be at the heart of all of the Public Health Service's efforts.[22] While the relationship of poverty to sexual behavior and teenage pregnancy is more complex than Elders' sound bites made it appear, her simplification of the issue had a broad appeal both to the many Americans who endorsed comprehensive sex education and the many public health experts who were eager to develop and implement concrete programs to address this issue.[23]

Those who wondered just how Elders would address the problems of sexually transmitted disease and teenage pregnancy had only to watch as she packed up her desk accessories to move from Little Rock to Washington, D.C. Among the most prominent items to make the journey was a bouquet of faux flowers made from condom wrappers. The bouquet, which had been given to Elders by a colleague and had long sat on her desk in Little Rock, had signs attached to it: "Blooms Mostly at Night . . . Blooms May Wilt in Chilly Atmosphere." One look at the bouquet, and the future of federally funded efforts to promote sex education was clear.[24]

Within the first four months of her appointment, Elders was everywhere. Appearing on the popular news show *This Week with David Brinkley*, she urged Americans to provide and support sex education in their schools. These efforts were, she insisted, central to reducing out-of-wedlock births. She publicly lamented what she called the nation's fear of sex. "I personally feel that the underlying issue is sex," she told a reporter. Linked to the nation's fear of sex was the belief that "fornication must be punished and that teenage pregnancy and the bad things that happen are the punishment." In January 1994 she followed up on this comment, pointing out that while "everyone in the world is opposed to sex outside of marriage . . . everyone does it." It was, she insisted, time to "Get Real." Elders' controversial comments on public health were not limited to sex education. She also spoke about the need to put health clinics in the nation's schools, the importance of reassessing the nation's drug policies, and the need to immunize and care for the nation's poor—all policies that had little or no appeal to those on the Far Right. But it was Elders' comments on sex education that sparked the most heated controversy. By the spring of her first year in office, Catholic bishops had condemned Elders' discussion of homosexuality as an attempt at a "re-definition of the family." Republicans in Congress had publicly called for her firing, and conservative and liberal columnists were building their careers on the Elders sound bite.[25]

In short, Elders fulfilled all of the expectations those on both the Left and the Right had had with regard to her appointment. As an admiring John Cowan, the co-founder of Lead or Leave, an advocacy group for adolescents, pointed out, the "political system is squeamish about the truth," but Elders was prepared to advocate for the truth "as far as young people are concerned." She is "the only person in [a] . . . high position who speaks about how gay and lesbian people live in this country and . . . [how] they are a part of communities," Robin Kane of the National Gay and Lesbian Task Force noted with pleasure. But others remained uneasy. While admitting that new ideas come from those who push at existing boundaries, Kent Amos of the Urban Institute worried that some of the surgeon general's comments "inflame passions and emotions that are not productive." This ability to antagonize her opponents had led even some who agreed with her to step back. Thomas Parrish, the pastor of a Lutheran church in rural Minnesota, noted ruefully that while he agreed with "about 85% of what she does," Elders' approach to public health was so abrasive that he had not hesitated to protest when she was invited to speak to religious leaders in his community.[26]

In 1987, when then–Arkansas governor Clinton had introduced Elders at a news conference, he had remarked with some amusement, "I know how Abraham Lincoln felt when he met Harriet Beecher Stowe [and he said]: This is the little lady that started the great war."[27] Elders' appointment as surgeon general had intensified the battle for sex education, and the attacks on comprehensive and abstinence-only programs now came from both the Left and the Right in a fast, furious, and almost constant barrage. Some of the criticism aimed at Elders and her calls for comprehensive sex education was, as both she and Clinton knew, part of a broader attack by Christian conservatives on Clinton himself. But Elders' refusal to tone down her rhetoric meant that by 1994 she had her own very vocal, and very active, group of detractors.[28]

Given both the doggedness with which those on the Right tracked every comment Elders made and Elders' own tendency to speak bluntly and off the cuff, it was just a matter of time before the controversy exploded. Fifteen months after her appointment, Elders' opponents found her Achilles heel when

Elders casually responded to a reporter's questions on World AIDS Day. Although Elders' exact response will never be known, the gist of her comments was enough to seal her fate. Asked by a psychologist in the audience if she believed that there would ever be a shift in the taboo against public discussions about masturbation as a component of human sexuality, Elders responded that she viewed masturbation as a natural part of human sexuality. Yes, she said firmly, she believed that discussions about masturbation should be included in sex education.

Proving that masturbation was indeed a taboo subject, a very public outcry quickly erupted. Calls for Elders' firing were, as they had always been, extraordinarily loud and persistent. This time Clinton, who found himself under growing attack by the Religious Right and even many on the Left, had little choice but to fire Elders. Within two weeks of her statement, Elders was out of a job. In an ironic twist that Elders must have later savored, those who led the call for her ouster—Bill Clinton and Newt Gingrich—would soon provide graphic illustrations of Elders' earlier remark that while "everyone is opposed to sex outside of marriage . . . everyone does it." But in December of 1994, all that was in the future.[29]

Elders' fall was in many ways predictable. Of all of Clinton's appointees, she had been the one who most enraged the Religious Right. The reasons for this antagonism are complex. The views of the Religious Right on race and gender cannot be neatly categorized, but the movement experienced its greatest growth during the push both to desegregate schools and to deny tax-exempt status to schools that segregate on the basis of race. Many members of the movement have also called for a return to the "traditional family," a call that may indicate some opposition to women in the workplace. Obviously not all members of the Religious Right endorse racist or sexist views, but the fact that the movement has often been most active on issues relating to race and gender, as well as the fact that leaders of the movement, such as Jerry Falwell, have openly advocated racist views, would seem to indicate a strong racist element in the movement. These factors meant that Elders was unacceptable as a surgeon general to many members of the Religious Right, simply because of her race and gender. But Elders' refusal to kowtow or even tone down her rhetoric when speaking to or about those on the Far Right really solidified their anger against her.[30] Many of the statements Elders made were no different from those made by Koop. But Koop, unlike Elders, had retained credibility among many moderates and even some on the Far Right. As a result, he had greater latitude to speak about sex education, and this greater latitude had been central to his longevity in office.

In the wake of Elders' fall, many Americans expressed discontent with Clinton's decision to fire her. From Parsippany, New Jersey, Joseph Wardy wrote to his local paper, pointing out that "taboos [against] masturbation remain taboos unless we fight them." From Boulder, Colorado, one columnist noted that in firing Elders, Clinton and Gingrich "were speaking in code, past me, and past most moderate Americans, to the religious far right." In Boston, Roger Gauthier told a reporter, "I liked her. I thought she was up-front but that was her problem apparently." From Iowa City, William Stosine pulled no punches. His letter to the editor followed Elders' own blunt approach: "Anyone who thinks she would advocate teaching a 'how-to' course in masturbation in schools is an idiot indoctrinated in conservative propaganda."[31]

If Elders' dismissal did little to assuage the concerns of the many Americans who were in favor of comprehensive sex education, it also did nothing to buy Clinton support among those on the Far Right. As Clinton would discover, the Religious Right was not prepared to negotiate a compromise on any of their core issues, nor were they prepared to temper their criticisms of Clinton himself.

"A Mainstream Physician"

Clinton's first choice for Elders' successor as surgeon general was Henry Foster, an African-American gynecologist and obstetrician. In the 1980s Foster had founded a comprehensive sex education program called "I Have a Future." The program, which had been implemented in the housing projects of Foster's home state of Tennessee, included tutoring, job training, and medical services. It also taught children about contraception. During the presidency of George H. W. Bush, Foster and his program had been recognized as one of the "thousand points of light," but when Clinton moved to nominate Foster, an outcry erupted among those on the Far Right.

The problem? As an obstetrician, Foster had performed abortions. The exact number of the abortions Foster had performed was never clarified, although it appeared to have been relatively low. While the media went for the quick sound bite and clearly enjoying playing up the tensions between those on the Far Left and those on the Far Right, Foster's views on abortion were complex. Like many of his fellow Americans, Foster viewed abortion as a last resort. Additionally, no evidence indicated that Foster had performed abortions before they became legal. But legal or not, Foster's actions in this regard were sufficient to damn him in the eyes of those on the Right. Warning that "the Senate Republican leadership needs to stop being so squeamish and . . . stand forthrightly behind the pro-life views they say they hold," James A. Smith, a leading lobbyist for the Southern Baptists, insisted that it was time for the "Senate Republican leadership to get engaged in the culture war." Denying their support for Foster's appointment would, Smith suggested, be a good start. Among Catholics, Foster also encountered opposition. Especially vocal in their opposition was a small group of African-American Catholics led by Dolores Bernadette Grier. Rejecting all attempts to shade the issue, Grier told her 500-member organization, "The man is not black. The man is not white. He is an abortionist who terminates life in the womb and that's what he should be judged by."[32]

In the weeks that followed, mounting opposition to Foster made it clear that he could not win the nomination, and Clinton, eager to avoid yet another showdown with the Religious Right, began to look for a less controversial candidate for surgeon general. In David Satcher, an African-American physician who had, like Elders, risen from extreme poverty to become the director of the Centers for Disease Control and Prevention, Clinton found a "mainstream physician who is an eloquent advocate for the health of all Americans." Although his nomination came under attack by Senator John Ashcroft, Satcher had overwhelming support among the majority of congressional legislators, and he was confirmed in February 1998.[33]

Satcher, as he well knew, was stepping into an oversized uniform. In interview after interview he told reporters, "I'm not Dr. Elders or Dr. Koop." But, he added, "I still have a lot to say in my own way." Firmly insisting that he wanted to be "the best David Satcher I can be," the new surgeon general found himself walking a fine line as he struggled both to find his own voice and to become the aggressive advocate for public health that he believed the nation needed.[34]

Unlike his immediate predecessor, Satcher was not one to court controversy. "The first thing that I am looking for," he told a reporter, "is agreement on where we want to go as a nation." But Satcher, who characterized himself as someone who "love[s] a good fight but . . . [doesn't] go out looking for one," quickly found that this approach raised problems, at least when it came to sex education. After a year in office a frustrated Satcher was forced to admit that the Religious Right "has opposed a lot of the things I've tried to do . . . to help people reduce their risk for HIV transmission." "I've tried," a weary Satcher confessed, to "work around them or work through them but I wouldn't dare say I've figured out how to deal with them yet."[35]

Compounding Satcher's problems was the Monica Lewinsky scandal, which erupted shortly after Satcher took office. As discussions of oral sex became common on the nightly news, Satcher found himself in an awkward position. Would an aggressive discussion of sex education and sexual responsibility simply compound his boss' problems? Tiptoeing his way through what had become a political minefield, Satcher found himself forced to weigh his words when speaking about sex education.

"We're Continuing That Tradition"

In 1998 Satcher had been appointed to a four-year term as Surgeon General. When a beleaguered Clinton left office in 2000, Satcher elected to remain in his position. Although there was little to indicate that the new president, George W. Bush, would support an activist surgeon general, Satcher clearly felt he had some unfinished business, specifically the release of a long-awaited surgeon general's report on American sexuality. Like Novello and Koop, Satcher had come to believe that these reports were one of the best ways of provoking a national discussion on sex education, and in the summer of 2001 Satcher released his own report, which was, he emphasized, "based on science."

With this report Satcher sought to explain once and for all why the nation needed to endorse and support comprehensive sex education programs. Sexually transmitted diseases infected approximately 12 million Americans each year. Over 700,000 new cases of AIDS had been reported since 1981. Nearly half of all pregnancies in the United States were unintended, and over a million abortions had been performed since 1996. "Each of these problems," the report stated, "carries with it the potential for lifelong consequences for individuals, families, communities and the nation as a whole." Calling for a "mature and thoughtful discussion about sexuality," Satcher admitted that asking Americans to find "common ground might not be easy," but it was essential if Americans were to "lay a foundation for a healthier society in the future." The time had come for Americans to get serious about promoting a comprehensive and nuanced program of sex education.[36]

At heart, *The Surgeon General's Call to Action to Promote Sexual Health and Responsible Sexual Behavior* did not advocate anything really new. Emphasizing the use of science, the report sought to clarify several key issues about sex, sexuality, and sex education. There was no scientific evidence indicating that comprehensive sex education led to early sexual activity. There was no scientific evidence that sexual orientation could be changed. There was no scientific evidence that abstinence-only education prevented or even delayed teens from having sex. Scientific studies did, however, indicate that a high incidence of sexually transmitted disease, unintended pregnancy, rape, and sexual abuse plagued the nation.

For those on the Left, the report was anticlimactic. "I yawn . . . over this report . . . the progressive elements are news only to the hopelessly clueless," snorted one columnist on the Left. A Seattle columnist agreed, pointing out that the report was "neither radical nor revolutionary." But even as those on the Left chided Satcher for failing to advocate a more aggressive approach to sex education, Satcher found himself under attack by the Bush administration and its constituents.[37]

Tommy Thompson, the secretary of the Department of Health and Human Services, quickly distanced himself from Satcher, insisting that *The Call to Action* was "independent work." Pointing out that the report had not been released during the Clinton administration, Bush's spokesperson Ari Fleischer maintained that the report had probably not been released because Clinton officials "must have seen something in it that would make them delay it." The delay in the report's release undoubtedly stemmed from Satcher's reluctance to release a report on sexual responsibility at a time when Clinton was undergoing an impeachment trial on charges of sexual irresponsibility. But for Fleischer and the many officials in the Bush administration who were reluctant to endorse or even appear to endorse Satcher's report, the delay provided a convenient excuse to condemn it.[38]

While there was little in the report that was news to the American people, the report did present problems for the Bush administration. The contested nature of Bush's presidency meant that he was heavily dependent on the right wing of his own party. And the Religious Right had, as both Bush and Satcher knew, long advocated the removal of comprehensive sex education programs from the nation's schools. In his *Call to Action* Satcher broke with both his predecessor, Antonia Novello, and his new boss, George W. Bush. Rather than advocating that the home should be the driving force behind sex education, Satcher called upon schools to become "the great equalizer." Pointing out what many Americans already knew, Satcher gently reminded his fellow citizens that parents routinely failed to provide their children with sex education. Satcher also noted that Americans overwhelming endorsed comprehensive sex education programs in schools. Wasn't it time, he asked, for American schools to fulfill their promise by providing American children with comprehensive sex education?[39]

But this was not the only element of Satcher's report that caused the Bush administration to distance itself from Satcher. Satcher's terse remarks about the lack of scientific evidence regarding the effectiveness of abstinence-only sex education won him no support among those who had spent decades advocating this type of education. Equally problematic was Satcher's strong statement that sexual orientation could not be altered. But even as he angered those on the Far Right, Satcher demonstrated that he was exactly what Clinton had promised: a "mainstream physician." By 2000 the majority of Americans accepted and agreed with these views on sex, sexuality, and sexual responsibility.

Yet even as Satcher did little to challenge mainstream America's views on sex education, the Bush administration was opting to follow a very different path. Eager to appease its constituents on the Far Right, the administration began a series of initiatives designed to alter American sex education. Many of these initiatives entailed a continuation and even escalation of policies that had begun under Reagan and that had continued under the first president Bush and Clinton. Other tactics were new.

In 1996, as part of the Clinton administration's welfare reform initiatives, Congress had agreed to provide $50 million annually to states that used abstinence-only sex education as the standard for schoolchildren. Matching funds, provided by the states, pushed this amount up to $87.5 million annually. The grant program provided a strong and clear definition for what constituted abstinence-only education. Abstinence-only education programs stressed the "social, psychological, and health gains" of remaining abstinent until marriage. They also promoted abstinence as the standard and only acceptable form of sexual behavior. Teachers in abstinence-only programs stated that abstinence was the only way to prevent pregnancies and sexually transmitted diseases; that monogamy within the context of marriage was the only acceptable form of sexual activity; that any type of sexual activity outside of marriage would have "harmful psychological and physical effects;" and that bearing children out of wedlock would have "harmful consequences for the child, the child's parents and society." Also emphasized were methods to teach young adults how to reject sexual advances. Educators stressed the importance of attaining self-sufficiency before engaging in sexual activity.[40]

From the perspective of those who advocated comprehensive sex education, this approach to sex education was riddled with problems. Children who are born out of wedlock are stigmatized by these programs, critics charged. Moreover, in a society that denies same-sex couples the right to marry, abstinence-only programs such as these imply that homosexuals and lesbians should never engage in consensual sex with same-sex partners. Worse yet, said many on the Left, abstinence-only programs "exaggerated the failure rate of condoms" and used "terror tactics to keep teens from having sex."[41] These criticisms had no effect on funding for abstinence-only programs. Between 1996 and 2005, $1 billion was channeled into abstinence-only programs.

What were Americans getting in exchange for the money? By 2005 the United States had the highest teenage pregnancy rate of any nation in the industrialized world. And yet Americans were no more or less sexually active than their counterparts in other industrialized nations.

The fault, Representative Henry Waxman charged, lay in the nation's approach to sex education. In 2004, two years after Satcher left office, researchers prepared a comprehensive report on sex education at Waxman's request. Focusing on the "most popular abstinence-only curricula used by grantees of the largest federal abstinence initiative," researchers discovered that over 80 percent of the curricula used by the majority of grantees contained "false, misleading or distorted information about reproductive health." The report also found that there had been a continuation of the blurring of religion and science that had plagued federally funded programs in the 1980s and 1990s. Many of these programs endorsed outdated gender stereotypes. The most notorious of these was a program called "Choosing the Best." Widely cited in the press, "Choosing the Best" featured a story in which a knight attempted to rescue a village from a dragon. At a loss as to how to kill the dragon, the knight receives advice from a princess. While the knight uses the advice to kill the dragon, his reliance on the princess leaves him feeling "ashamed." Rather than marry the princess, he chooses instead to marry a village maiden "after making sure she knew nothing" about how to kill a dragon. The moral of the story? Too much advice "will lessen a man's confidence and turn him away from his princess." The story and its use in an abstinence-only curriculum graphically demonstrated the complex agenda of many of those who advocated abstinence-only programs.[42]

But it was the disregard for science that most angered Waxman. Looking at these and other curricula, a frustrated Waxman said, "I have no objection [to] talking [about] abstinence as a surefire way to prevent unwanted pregnancy and sexually transmitted diseases . . . [but] I don't think we ought to lie to our children about science." Something, he concluded, "is seriously wrong when federal tax dollars are being used to mislead kids about basic health facts."

In response to Waxman's report, the Bush administration was quick to defend itself. Even though Waxman had indicated that he had "no objection" to talking about "abstinence as a surefire way to prevent" pregnancy and disease, Alma Golden, the assistant deputy secretary for population affairs in the Department of Health and Human Services, moved quickly to imply that Waxman did not support abstinence. The report, Golden lamented in the press, did "a disservice to our children." In a statement that Waxman would have, and in fact already had, endorsed, Golden reminded her fellow Americans that abstinence is "the most effective means of preventing the sexual transmission of HIV, STDs and preventing pregnancy." Golden's approach was nothing new; both opponents and proponents of comprehensive sex education had spent the last three decades speaking past one another in this fashion.[43]

But problems were not limited to how federal dollars were being used to promote abstinence-only programs. The surgeon general who replaced Satcher, Richard Carmona, proved reluctant to voice his opposition to the Bush administration's policies on sex education. While Carmona later claimed that he had been expressly forbidden to express his views on sex education, his unwillingness to speak publicly did little to counter the administration's reluctance to "hear the science."[44] This disregard for science was especially troubling as the science on sex education was becoming clearer.

By 2007 the mainstream media began publicizing facts that scientists, statisticians, and public health experts had long suspected. Teens in abstinence-only programs not only engage in sex, they are also less likely to use protection than their peers who receive comprehensive sex education. While religious belief strongly correlates with attitudes toward sexual activity (evangelical teens, for example, are more likely than nonevangelicals to say that they will abstain from sex outside of marriage), it is not always a strong predictor of sexual activity. On average, white teens who identify themselves as evangelicals become sexually active shortly after turning sixteen; their white peers who define themselves as Jews, mainline Protestants, Catholics, or Mormons not only become sexually active at a later age, they are less sexually active than evangelical teens. But even this finding needs to be nuanced; teens who attend church regularly and who strongly identify with their evangelical beliefs tend to be less sexually active than their fellow evangelicals who are not as religiously active. Reflecting this pattern of behavior, the states in the Bible Belt are generally more likely to have

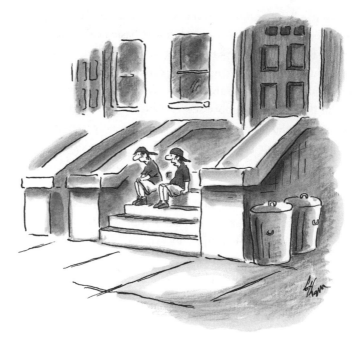

"I was an abstinence-only baby."

The failure of abstinence-only education programs to prevent pregnancy quickly came to be seen as a joke (2008). *The New Yorker.* © The New Yorker Collection 2008 Frank Cotham from cartoonbank.com. All rights reserved.

high rates of teen pregnancy than their counterparts elsewhere. However, it is unclear whether public health experts were focusing on the right factors when assessing teenagers' sexual behavior.[45]

Throughout both Bush administrations, the Public Health Service and its parent, the Department of Health and Human Services, provided few opportunities to those who were eager to explore and candidly discuss the factors influencing teens' sexual behavior or the best ways to prevent sexually transmitted diseases and unwanted pregnancies.[46] Newspaper reports also indicate that the administration of George W. Bush may have been directly involved in activities ranging from rewriting federally funded websites on sexual health to repeatedly auditing organizations that advocate comprehensive sex education.[47] Lawsuits have also been filed alleging that federal funds have been used to promote religion in federally funded abstinence-only programs.[48]

Chilling as these actions may have been to those who advocate an open discussion about sex education, George W. Bush administration's very aggressive attempts to limit the debate on sex education had an unforeseen effect. By advocating a one-size-fits-all sex education message, the administration united a diverse and growing number of Americans, all of whom believed that sex education should be both comprehensive and secular.

"Individual Responsibility and Mutual Responsibility"

In the summer of 2008, as the presidential election heated up, the McCain campaign released a thirty-second ad attacking Senator Barack Obama. "Obama's one accomplishment?" the ad asked. "Legislation to teach kindergarteners comprehensive sex education." Within days, fact-checking organizations and the media had released assessments of the ad. Pointing out that Obama had called for "age-appropriate sex education" for young children, pundits and columnists quickly agreed that the ad was "off-base" and a distortion of Obama's stance on sex education.[49] Left undiscussed in these assessments was the fact that Obama's stance on sex education differed little from the position proposed by the federal government ninety years earlier.[50] But the rush to clarify Obama's position on sex education reflected the fact that sex education still remained a hot-button issue across the United States. And while it quickly became clear that the McCain campaign had distorted Obama's position, the ad graphically illustrated how discussions about sex education can be and often are used both to stoke the culture wars and to advance very different political agendas.

Obama's own views on both sex education and the nature of discussions about sexually active teens were clearly articulated throughout his campaign. When news of Bristol Palin's pregnancy broke, Obama issued a withering condemnation of those who sought to make the story an issue. Reminding Americans that his own mother had been both a teenager and pregnant when she married his father, Obama insisted that "how a family deals with issues and teenage children . . . shouldn't be the topic of our politics, and . . . if I ever thought that there was somebody in my campaign that was involved in [exploiting] something like that, they'd be fired."[51] For Obama, the broader issue was not about the pregnancies of high-profile teens—or even how the actions of high-profile teens could be used as focal points in broader political debates—but rather about how Americans deal with the issue overall. In his acceptance speech at the Democratic National Convention in August 2008, Obama sought to find and to remind his fellow citizens of the common ground that many Americans hold in regard to sex education. "We may not all agree on abortion," he said, "but we can all agree we want to reduce the number of abortions." For many Americans, Obama's comments were a clarion call for the nation to provide better sex education. But even as Americans on both sides of the aisle nodded in approval of this measured statement, Obama's comments in Denver sparked protests at his campaign headquarters in the nearby and heavily evangelical city of Colorado Springs.[52]

Clearly there were to be no easy answers to the questions of how and why sex education should be taught.

EPILOGUE

Dear Beth," the letter read, "sex education should not be taught in schools. Children should learn from their parents. . . . When the subject is discussed in schools, children learn that sex is something they should start right away." For the advice columnist who received this letter, the answer was clear: "Teachers who are properly trained do an excellent job" of providing sex education. More important, the columnist gently pointed out, "there is no indication that sex education leads to increased sexual activity."[1] The letter and its response appeared in the *Boston Globe* in 1987, but it could have appeared in 1927 or even 2007.

Since the Public Health Service launched its first sex education campaign in 1918, discussions about sex education, its uses, and its limits have been a constant in American society. Over the past ninety years these discussions have been remarkably consistent. In 1918, parents, employers, teachers, and even adolescents themselves called for government-sponsored sex education. Today the situation is little different. As recently as 2000 a Kaiser Family Foundation study revealed that an overwhelming majority of Americans are still calling for more aggressive sex education. They are also expressing deep concerns about the spread of sexually transmitted diseases and the rise in teenage pregnancies.

Despite these commonalities, public debates about sex education have become increasingly heated over the last forty years. Some of this controversy stems from the diverse nature of American society. But much of it stems from our profound uneasiness with the idea of adolescents engaging in sex. As we struggle with this anxiety and differing views on sex, we often ignore certain unpleasant facts about our past. Since the founding of Jamestown in 1607, significant percentages of teenagers and young adults have engaged in premarital sex.[2] But acknowledging this truth still leaves us with the troubling fact that the age at which teens become sexually active has dropped steadily since the 1970s. Today, over half of all teenagers are sexually active by the age of nineteen. Numerous scientific studies have explored the different reasons why teens become sexually active, and the mainstream media and different organizations have all rushed to point accusatory fingers at factors ranging from sexually explicit television to working parents.

Unfortunately this reluctance to acknowledge and speak candidly about our sexual behavior has shaped our views on sex education. In Osseo, Minnesota, a sixteen-year-old sophomore typifies the nation's reluctance to engage in an honest discussion about sex, abstinence, monogamy and contraception. "I've always known I would save sex for marriage. It's just the way I was brought up," the teenager earnestly told a reporter. Given a choice as to whether she would take a comprehensive sex education class or one that advocated abstinence-only, she opted for an abstinence-only class. Her choice to take the class and her public decision to remain abstinent would have been admirable "had her best friend not mentioned the day before that this same girl had just gone through a terrifying two-and-a-half month pregnancy scare."[3] Throughout the twentieth century, public health experts, parents, and writers ranging from Upton Sinclair to Judy Blume have explored the problems that occur when teenagers and young adults fail, as this Minnesotan did, to follow the path of abstinence. These failures have provided wonderful fodder for films such as *Juno*, *The Graduate*, and *The End of the Road*, for the pulp fiction of the 1930s and books such as the teen classic *Forever*, for television shows such as *James at Fifteen* and *The Gilmore Girls*, and even for plays such as *Damaged Goods* and *Blue Denim*. But for the federal government, the choices of these fictional figures have presented a minefield when acted out by real teens in places like Osseo, Minnesota.

In negotiating this minefield, the Public Health Service has preferred to err on the side of caution when creating sex education programs. More often than not, federally funded sex education campaigns have endorsed conservative views of sex that are at odds with Americans' sexual behavior. In the early years of the twentieth century, this approach was problematic, but it was to some degree understandable. Early-twentieth-century Americans wanted the government to provide sex education, but they were also uneasy about having federal officials step into the nation's bedrooms. Conservative sex education programs have gone a long way toward reassuring Americans that the government would not overstep its boundaries or force them to acknowledge unpleasant truths about their own behavior.

In recent years this push toward conservatism has led to abstinence-only education programs becoming more common. As their problems have become increasingly apparent, detailed and rigorous studies of these programs have indicated what many public health experts have long feared. At a cost of $1 billion over the last ten years, these programs have routinely presented students with scientifically inaccurate information while endorsing strangely outdated and irrelevant gender stereotypes. Troubling as these problems are, the failure of these programs to reshape teens' sexual behavior has provoked the greatest outcry among public health experts. A stunning 88 percent of teens who took abstinence-only pledges nevertheless engaged in sex before marriage. Teens in abstinence-only programs had the same rates of sexually transmitted disease as those who had attended comprehensive sex education programs. Most chilling, however, was the discovery that teens in abstinence-only programs were less likely to use condoms than their peers in comprehensive programs, and they were less likely to see a doctor when they contracted a sexually transmitted disease than their peers who had attended comprehensive sex education programs. Abstinence-only programs were, in other words, ineffective at preventing teens from engaging in sex outside of marriage, and they were also compounding the problem of sexually transmitted diseases by facilitating their spread.[4]

Shortly after the presidential election in 2004, Wade Horn, the assistant secretary for children and families in the Department of Health and Human Services, had announced that "we don't need a study" on the effectiveness of abstinence-only sex education programs. "Those people who are sexually abstinent have a zero chance of becoming pregnant or getting someone pregnant or contracting a sexually transmitted disease," Horn stated.[5] But Horn's views are those of a minority. Increasingly states are distancing themselves from the federal government on this issue. In late 2007, fourteen states decided to forgo millions of dollars in federal funding so that they could regain the right to provide their students with comprehensive sex education programs, as opposed to abstinence-only programs.[6]

As states increasingly agree to forgo federal funds for their sex education programs and as the federal government advocates an approach to sex education at odds with the views of most Americans, two key questions remain. After nearly one hundred years of providing Americans with sex education, will the efforts of the federal government in providing Americans with information on sex become increasingly irrelevant? And if so, what will the consequences be for the vast majority of Americans who have depended on the federal government to provide them with the sex education they need and want?

NOTES

ONE: In Bed with the Fed

1. "A Case of Too Much Candor," *US News and World Report*, December 19, 1994, p. 31; Douglas Jehl, "Surgeon General Forced to Resign by White House," *New York Times*, December 9, 1994, p. 1.

2. Claudia Dreifus, "Joycelyn Elders," *New York Times Magazine*, January 30, 1994, p. 16.

3. For a discussion of this unease, see Theda Skocpol, "A Society without a 'State'? Political Organization, Social Conflict, and Welfare Provision," *Journal of Public Policy*, vol. 7, no. 6 (October–December 1987), pp. 368–369.

4. Kimberley S. Johnson, *Governing the American State* (Princeton: Princeton University Press, 2006), p. 6.

5. Ronald Reagan, "Remarks at a Luncheon for Members of the College of Physicians in Philadelphia Pennsylvania," April 1, 1987.

6. "Continuing American ambivalence about the role of the state in social provision focuses most acutely on public programs for the poor and for blacks . . . vulnerable groups do best when bureaucrats and national political parties have worked together to build universal systems of public social provision, stretching from the upper middle classes to the poor . . . [but] US state structures have rarely allowed such coalitions to shape social policies." Skocpol, "Society without a 'State,'" p. 369.

7. William J. Novak, "The Myth of the 'Weak' American State," *American Historical Review*, June 2008, p. 763. Richard John also points out that historians "have neglected the role of the central government as an agent of change." Richard John, *Spreading the News: The American Postal System from Franklin to Morse* (Cambridge, Mass.: Harvard University Press, 1995), p. 18.

8. "An Act for the Relief of Sick and Disabled Seamen," 1 Stat. 605, Fifth Congress, 1797–1798.

9. "Max Edling, for example, has recently re-centered the history of the American founding around the creation of a strong 'fiscal-military' state . . . Jerry Mashaw has similarly traced the origins of a powerful and centralizing national administrative law to the first days of the republic, challenging the historical fiction that a national bureaucracy and administrative regulatory authority awaited the invention of the Interstate Commerce Commission." Novak, "Myth of the 'Weak' American State," p. 758.

10. For a complete discussion of this revolution and its impact on America, see Nancy Tomes, *The Gospel of Germs: Men, Women, and the Microbe in American Life* (Cambridge, Mass.: Harvard University Press, 1998).

11. Alexandra M. Lord, "Dangerous Waters: Washington DC, the Public Health Service, and the Typhoid Epidemic of 1906," unpublished paper delivered at the National Institutes of Health, Bethesda, Md., 2004.

12. This was not because researchers sought to keep the project a secret but rather because it was reported on only sporadically in public health and medical journals. James H. Jones, *Bad Blood: The Tuskegee Syphilis Experiment* (New York: Free Press, 1981), p. 7.

13. The CDC also actively campaigned to promote specific public health messages on different television shows. Sheryl Gay Stolberg, "CDC Plays Script Doctor to Spread Its Message," *New York Times*, June 26, 2001; Steve Sternberg, "AIDS Drives Plots on TV," *USA Today*, August 7, 2006. Television shows on which the CDC has played a prominent role range from *Law and Order*, "Patient Zero" (episode E4301, original airdate in North America October 8, 2003), to *House*, "Euphoria, Part II" (episode 221, original airdate in North America May 3, 2006.) The pilot episode of *The West Wing* delivered a double whammy for the CDC: a subplot involving the Christian Right provided an opening for a brief discussion of the CDC and its sex education programs. *The West Wing*, "Pilot" (episode 1, original airdate in North America September 22, 1999). Ironically, CDC missed out on its greatest publicity coup with *Medical Investigators*, a short-lived show on NBC (2005) that featured a government agency dedicated to tracking diseases and preventing epidemics; the show identified that agency as NIH, not CDC. While noting that "folks at CDC were not happy" about this mischaracterization, officials at NIH justified their cooperation with the show's producers by saying, "You can't buy publicity like that." The show failed to last more than one season. Carla Garnet, "Prime Time Show Offers NIH Opportunity," *NIH Record*, October 18, 2005.

14. Peter Baldwin, "The Scandinavian Origins of the Social Interpretation of the Welfare State," *Comparative Studies in Society and History*, vol. 31, no. 1 (January 1989), pp. 3–24.

15. Jim Shahin, "Flying the Koop," *American Way Magazine*, June 15, 1989, p. 62.

16. *The Simpsons*, "Homer's Barbershop Quartet" (episode 9F21, original airdate in North America September 30, 1993). Koop also appeared on another episode of *The Simpsons*, "Bye, Bye Nerdie" (episode CABF1, original airdate in North America March 11, 2001). Although Koop was not averse to appearing in films and, although the producers of *The Simpsons* have often recruited public figures such as Tony Blair, Stephen Hawking, and Stephen Jay Gould to play themselves on air, Koop did not do the voice-over for the Koop character.

17. *The Colbert Report*, "The Word: Pathophysiology" (episode 272, original airdate in North America June 13, 2007); *The Daily Show*, "You Have No Idea!" (episode 12090, original airdate in North America July 17, 2007); *The Daily Show*, "Chain Smoke" (episode 3107, original airdate in North America March 16, 1999).

18. By 1981 a substantial number of the hospitals owned by the Public Health Service had already been closed. While the reasons for the hospitals' closure were complex, it is clear that many conservatives disliked the idea of merchant marines receiving federally subsidized health care.

19. This ability to police Americans' sexual behavior predated the nation's founding; colonial governments had routinely passed laws criminalizing certain sexual activities, and while the criminalization of contraception and abortion was not consistent during this period, state governments did pass legislation limiting or even forbidding these practices.

20. Ruth Rosen points to the period between 1850 and 1900 as seeing a peak in prostitution. In a society that prohibited women from engaging in sex outside of marriage and that often encouraged men to delay marriage, prostitutes filled an important role. Ruth Rosen, *The Lost Sisterhood: Prostitution in America, 1900–1918* (Baltimore: Johns Hopkins University Press, 1982), p. 3.

21. According to the reformer Florence Kelly, dance halls were "a constant menace to the moral security of those who frequent them." F. Kelly, "Some Causes of Prostitution," *Women's Medical Journal*, vol. 20 (1910), p. 38. For a broad discussion of dating patterns during this period, see Mary Odem, *Delinquent Daughters: Protecting and Policing Adolescent Female Sexuality in the United States, 1885–1920* (Chapel Hill: University of North Carolina Press, 1995); Kathy Peiss, *Cheap Amusements: Working Women and Leisure in Turn of the Century New York* (Philadelphia: University of Pennsylvania Press, 1986); and Beth Bailey, *From Front Porch Swing to Back Seat: Courtship in Twentieth-Century America* (Baltimore: Johns Hopkins University Press, 1988).

22. See, for example, Katherine Blee, *Women of the Klan: Racism and Gender in the 1920s* (Berkeley: University of California Press, 1992).

23. Theda Skocpol, *Social Policy in the United States: Future Possibilities in Historical Perspective* (Princeton: Princeton University Press, 1995), pp. 114–129.

24. Rachelle Yarros quoted in Regina Morantz-Sanchez, *Sympathy and Science: Women Physicians in American Medicine* (Oxford: Oxford University Press, 1985), p. 285.

25. Prince Morrow, the leader of the American Social Hygiene Association, believed that the "question of social hygiene [sex education] is a woman's question." "Society Reports: The Women's Medical Association of New York City [Meeting] Held at the Academy of Medicine, January 19, 1910," *Women's Medical Journal*, vol. 20 (1910), p. 44.

26. Skocpol, *Social Policy in the United States*, p. 9.

27. Federal expenditures on sex education have reflected the broad pattern of the government's expansion. Expenditures have spiked during crisis points such as the Depression and World War II, periods when the federal government grew.

28. Throughout most of the twentieth century, the majority of Americans have wanted sex education to be taught in schools.

29. Skocpol, *Social Policy in the United States*, p. 29.

30. Miriam Cohen and Michael Hanagn, "The Politics of Gender and the Making of the Welfare State, 1900–1940: A Comparative Perspective," *Journal of Social History*, vol. 24, no. 3 (Spring 1991), p. 473.

31. Of course, these different types of missions have blurred at times. In its early years Planned Parenthood reflected the eugenicist philosophy of its founder, Margaret Sanger. Its proponents aggressively sought to discourage the poor and the unfit from reproducing. But this approach did little to endear the organization to the poor, and by midcentury Planned Parenthood and similar organizations had come to serve an overwhelmingly white population.

32. Jeffrey Moran, *Teaching Sex: The Shaping of Adolescence in the Twentieth Century* (Cambridge, Mass.: Harvard University Press, 2002), pp. 178–183.

33. Simone M. Caron, "Birth Control and the Black Community in the 1960s," *Journal of Social History*, vol. 31, no. 3 (Spring 1998), pp. 545–569.

34. *The Problem of Sex Education in Schools* (Washington, D.C.: Public Health Service, 1918), p. 3.

35. Allan Brandt, *No Magic Bullet: A Social History of Venereal Disease in the United States since 1880* (Oxford: Oxford University Press, 1987), pp. 98, 107.

TWO: The People's War, 1918–1926

1. *A People's War* (Washington, D.C.: Public Health Service, 1919), pp. 5, 12.
2. Sinclair Lewis, *Babbit* (New York: Harcourt, Brace, Jovanovich, 1922; rpt. 1961), p. 74.
3. "Sex O'Clock in America," *Current Opinion*, August 1913, pp. 114–115.
4. The use of Salvarsan has varied over time. John Parascandola notes that in the period surrounding World War I, a "pharmacology textbook of the period described a typical treatment regimen as involving three doses of Salvarsan (or the more soluble related compound Neosalvarsan), generally administered by intravenous injection, given over a period of several weeks, followed by treatment with mercury. The author noted that this course of therapy might also have to be repeated at intervals until a permanent cure was effected." Twenty years later, treatment periods became even more extended. John Parascandola, *Sex, Sin, and Science: A History of Syphilis in America* (Westport, Conn.: Praeger, 2008), pp. 57–58, 77–78.
5. Upton Sinclair, *Damaged Goods* (Philadelphia: John C. Winston Co., 1913), p. 51.
6. *The Parents' Part* (Washington, D.C.: Public Health Service, 1918), pp. 8, 13.
7. "War on the Red Plague," *Daily Courier*, December 17, 1918. This article was reprinted in newspapers such as the *Middletown Daily Times Press*.
8. Andrea Tone, *Devices and Desires: A History of Contraceptives in America* (New York: Hill and Wang), pp. 67–159.
9. Parascandola, *Sex, Sin, and Science*, p. 49.
10. George Walker, *Venereal Diseases in the American Expeditionary Forces* (Baltimore: Medical Standard Book Co., 1922), p. 45.
11. For a full discussion of *Fit to Fight*, see Allan M. Brandt, *No Magic Bullet: A Social History of Venereal Disease in the United States since 1880* (Oxford: Oxford University Press, 1987), pp. 68–69, and Eric Schaefer, "Of Hygiene and Hollywood: Origins of the Exploitation Film," in *Hollywood: Critical Concepts in Media and Cultural Studies*, ed. Thomas Schatz (London: Routledge, 2003), pp. 169–171.
12. Parascandola, *Sex, Sin, and Science*, p. 57.
13. See, for example, Mary Odem, *Delinquent Daughters: Protecting and Policing Adolescent Female Sexuality, 1885–1920* (Chapel Hill: University of North Carolina Press, 1995), and Kathy Peiss, *Cheap Amusements: Working Women and Leisure in Turn of the Century New York* (Philadelphia: University of Pennsylvania Press, 1986).
14. "No Compromise with Prostitution!" *Fort Wayne News and Sentinel*, April 29, 1919.
15. "New Venereal Disease Law," *Evening Courier and Reporter*, June 7, 1919.
16. "War on the Red Plague."
17. "No Compromise with Prostitution"; *The Venereal Disease Handbook for Community Leaders* (Washington, D.C.: Public Health Service, 1924), p. 7.
18. Lewis, *Babbit*, p. 74; *The Problem of Sex Education in Schools* (Washington, D.C.: Public Health Service, 1918), p. 4.
19. C. C. Pierce to AA Surgeon D. J. Jacobson, 22 April, 1919, State Board of Health

file, Iowa folder, box 279, National Archives, College Park, Md.; "Health Picture at Englert's Theater," *Iowa City Citizen*, March 28, 1919.

20. Theodore Blank, "An Historical Survey of the Development of the Use of Audio-Visual Materials in Venereal Disease Education Programs, 1900–1949," Ph.D. diss., Boston University, 1970, p. 316. *Some Wild Oats* was seen in some small communities such as Elyria, Ohio. See "Some Wild Oats," *Chronicle Telegram*, September 22, 1920. In Iowa, the showing of the film was contested. See "Bar Wild Oats Film from Showing in Des Moines Picture House," *Evening Courier and Reporter*, September 20, 1921.

21. Karl S. Lashley and John B. Watson, "A Psychological Study of Motion Pictures in Relation to Venereal Disease Campaigns," *Journal of Social Hygiene*, vol. 2, no. 2 (1921), p. 181.

22. Newspaper excerpt [undated but from 1919], State Board of Health file, West Virginia folder, box 283, National Archives, College Park, Md.; Earl W. Brandenburg to J. A. Van Dis, May 29, 1919, YMCA file, Wisconsin folder, box 283, National Archives, College Park, Md.

23. *Two Years Fighting V.D.: A Report of the First Two Years' Work in the Program of Combating Venereal Diseases* (Washington, D.C.: Public Health Service, 1920), p. 14.

24. Theda Skocpol, *Social Policy in the United States: Future Possibilities in Historical Perspective* (Princeton: Princeton University Press, 1995), pp. 117–119. See also Alexandra M. Lord, "'Naturally Clean and Wholesome:' Women, Sex Education, and the United States Public Health Service, 1918–1928," *Social History of Medicine*, vol. 17, no. 3 (Winter 2004), pp. 423–441.

25. Julian B. Carter, *The Heart of Whiteness: Normal Sexuality and Race in America, 1880–1940* (Durham, N.C.: Duke University Press, 2007), p. 121.

26. Christina Simmons, "African Americans and Sexual Victorianism in the Social Hygiene Movement, 1910–1940," *Journal of the History of Sexuality*, vol. 4, no. 1 (July 1993), p. 55.

27. See, for example, Steven J. Hoffman, "Progressive Public Health Administration in the Jim Crow South: A Case Study of Richmond, Virginia, 1907–1920," *Journal of Social History*, vol. 35, no. 1 (Autumn 2001), p. 175.

28. See Sheena Morrison, "Beyond the Pale: National Negro Health Week and the Public Health Service," Ph.D. diss., Columbia University, forthcoming, and Simmons, "African Americans and Sexual Victorianism."

29. Charles V. Roman quoted in Simmons, "African Americans and Sexual Victorianism," p. 64.

30. *Two Years Fighting V.D.*, p. 23.

31. Michael Gold, *Jews without Money* (New York: Horace Liveright, 1930), p. 15.

32. Betty Smith, *A Tree Grows in Brooklyn* (1943; New York: Harper Perennial Classics, 1998), p. 246.

33. *Two Years Fighting V.D.*, p. 25.

34. Alexandra M. Lord, "Models of Masculinity: Sex Education, the United States Public Health Service, and the YMCA, 1919–1924," *Journal of the History of Medicine and Allied Sciences*, vol. 58, no. 2 (April 2003), p. 140.

35. "Secretary E. Lockman Addresses Boys at Phantom Lake," *Waukesha Freeman*, July 14, 1921.

36. C. Howard Hopkins, *History of the YMCA in North America* (New York: Associa-

tion Press, 1951), p. 385–386; Nancy Bristow, *Making Men Moral: Social Engineering during the Great War* (New York: New York University Press, 1996), p. 33.

37. *Problem of Sex Education in Schools*, p. 4.

38. *Two Years Fighting V.D.*, p. 11.

39. Ibid., p. 12.

40. "State boards of health were dubious about going ahead on account of the political situation and the Catholic element." J. A. Van Dis to E. M. Robinson, 22 April, 1919, E. M. Robinson file, Van Dis correspondence folder, box 288, National Archives and Records Administration, College Park, Md.

41. For a broader discussion of this approach and its relationship to privately funded sex education programs, see Carter, *Heart of Whiteness*, pp. 128–133.

42. National Keeping Fit Campaign, Miscellaneous folder, box 286, National Archives and Records Administration, College Park, Md.

43. YMCA Annual Report of J. A. Van Dis, marked Confidential, March 1, 1920, box 288, Personal file, National Archives, College Park, Md.

44. PHS officer Charles Claude Pierce, who headed the Public Health Service's Venereal Disease Division, admitted that "the real effect of ... [venereal disease] programs can never be known." C. C. Pierce, "Venereal Disease Control: Methods, Obstacles, and Results," *American Journal of Public Health*, vol. 10, no. 2 (1920), pp. 135–136.

45. *Two Years Fighting V.D.*, p. 19; "Social Diseases Rampant in State," *Ada Weekly News*, July 17, 1919.

46. *People's War*, pp. 14–15.

47. *Two Years Fighting V.D.*

48. Report from Arkansas, Biennial Report of the Department of Public Welfare, 1926–1928, General Federation of Women's Clubs Archives, Washington, D.C.

49. In 1919, 31.2 percent of American adolescents attended high school. By 1929, the number had jumped to 50.7 percent. David L. Angus and Jeffrey E. Mirrel, *The Failed Promise of the American High School, 1890–1995* (New York: Teachers College Press of Columbia University, 1999), p. 203.

50. "Sex O'Clock in America," p. 114.

51. *Manpower* (Washington, D.C.: Public Health Service, 1919), p. 15.

THREE: Battling the Mad Dog, 1927–1940

1. Perry Paul, "The Jane from Hell's Kitchen," in *Hard-Boiled Dames*, ed. Bernard Drew (New York: St. Martin's, 1986), pp. 234–235. The story was originally published in 1930.

2. Beth Bailey, *From Front Porch to Back Seat: Courtship in Twentieth-Century America* (Baltimore: Johns Hopkins University Press, 1988).

3. Robert Lynd and Helen Merrell Lynd, *Middletown: A Study in Modern American Culture* (New York: Harcourt and Brace, 1929), p. 140.

4. Graeme and Sara Lorimer, *First Love Farewell* (Boston: Little, Brown and Co., 1940), p. 74; Graeme and Sarah Lorimer, *Stag Line* (Boston: Little, Brown and Co., 1934), p. 7. In addition to the five Maudie books the Lorimers published during the 1930s, Maudie stories also appeared in the *Ladies Home Journal*. Maudie appeared on *Maudie's Diary* (CBS Radio) during the 1940s.

5. *Proceedings of Conference on Venereal Disease Control Work, Washington DC, December 28–30, 1936* (Washington, D.C.: Public Health Service, 1937), p. 19.

6. Ballard C. Campbell, "Federalism, State Action, and 'Critical Episodes' in the Growth of American Government," *Social Science History*, vol. 16, no. 4 (Winter 1992), pp. 561–577.

7. The PHS believed that venereal diseases rates were proportionately more prevalent in rural areas than in urban areas. "Biggest Problem," *Time*, January 27, 1936.

8. "Great Pox," *Time*, October 26, 1936.

9. The PHS had traditionally counted the number of sex education materials distributed as evidence of success. From the late 1940s on, the CDC's aggressive tracking of venereal disease and illegitimate pregnancies would force the PHS to be more honest in its assessment of its sex education programs.

10. Testimony of Dr. Felix Underwood, *Hearings before a Subcommittee of the Committee on Commerce, United States Senate, Seventy-fifth Congress, Third Session on S. 3290. A Bill to Impose Additional Duties upon the United States Public Health Service in Connection with the Investigation and Control of the Venereal Diseases*, February 14 and 15, 1938 (Washington, D.C., 1938), pp. 22–24.

11. For a full discussion of Underwood's career, see Lucie Robertson Bridgforth, "The Politics of Public Health Reform: Felix J. Underwood and the Mississippi State Board of Health, 1924–1958," *Public Historian*, vol. 6, no. 3 (Summer 1984), pp. 5–26.

12. Title VI of the Social Security Act dealt with public health. Section 601 of the Act stated, "For the purpose of assisting States, counties, health districts and other political subdivisions of the States in establishing and maintaining adequate public health service . . . there is hereby authorized to be appropriated for each fiscal year, beginning with the fiscal year ending June 30, 1936, the sum of $8,000,000."

13. Parran had actually asked for much more money to be dispersed over a ten-year period, but when it passed, the Act made only $15 million available over a three-year period. Funds became widely available in 1940.

14. Testimony of Mrs. Bauernschmidt, *Hearings . . . on S. 3290*, p. 18.

15. "Ladies and Syphilis," *Time*, July 19, 1937.

16. "Syphilis and Radio," *Time*, December 3, 1934.

17. "Biggest Problem."

18. Frank Nugent, "Dr. Ehrlich's Magic Bullet," *New York Times*, February 24, 1940.

19. "Great Pox."

20. Alan Brandt, *No Magic Bullet: A Social History of Venereal Disease in the United States since 1880* (Oxford: Oxford University Press, 1986), p. 142.

21. Several newspapers bragged that they had been using the word *syphilis* since the early 1920s. The *Chicago Tribune*, for example, claimed to have used the word as early as 1921. Suzanne Poirier, *Chicago's War on Syphilis: The Times, the Trib, and the Clap Doctor* (Champaign-Urbana: University of Illinois Press, 1995), p. 11. The PHS was well aware that newspapers all over the United States used these terms. See *Two Years Fighting Venereal Disease* (Washington, D.C.: Public Health Service, 1921), p. 7. See also "Great Pox."

22. Thomas Parran, Speech Given on Receipt of the Snow Medal for Distinguished Service, February 3, 1939, Personnel Records of Thomas Parran, Office of the Public Health Service Historian, Rockville, Md.

23. "Great Pox."

24. "Venereal Disease Campaign," *Time*, January 11, 1937.

25. Christina Simmons, "African Americans and Sexual Victorianism in the Social Hygiene Movement, 1910–1940," *Journal of the History of Sexuality*, vol. 4, no. 1 (July 1993), pp. 64–67.

26. Elizabeth Fee, "Sin vs. Science: Venereal Disease in Twentieth-Century Baltimore," in *AIDS: The Burdens of History*, ed. Elizabeth Fee and Daniel Fox (Berkeley: University of California Press, 1988), pp. 121–143.

27. As Fee points out, the belief that African Americans were inherently promiscuous was deeply rooted in American culture at this time. Even the residents of northern cities clung to this misconception. It should be no surprise, then, that public health officials in Baltimore, which straddled North and South, developed policies that reflected these views. Ibid. The sponsors of National Negro Health Week worked with the PHS on a variety of different public health projects at this time. See Sheena Morrison, "Beyond the Pale: Public Health Reform and the American Negro, 1895–1950," Ph.D. diss., Columbia University, forthcoming.

28. Gilbert Sandler, *Small Town Baltimore: An Album of Memories* (Baltimore: Johns Hopkins University Press, 2002), p. 22.

29. Testimony of Mrs. Bauernschmidt, *Hearings . . . on S. 3290*, p. 18.

30. Ibid.

31. The unique nature of Washington, D.C., which is located outside the jurisdiction of any state authority, made PHS officials reluctant to use the city or its experiences when exploring any public health problem. Located only thirty-five miles north of Washington, Baltimore was easily accessible by PHS officers, even those stationed in D.C.

32. This translated to one clinic per 130,000 people; this was an improvement over the national average of one clinic per 150,000. The study cited here was done in 1935. R. A. Vonderlehr, "Relationship of the Public Health Service to the Program for the Control of Syphilis and Gonorrhea in Greater New York," *Public Health Reports*, vol. 51, no. 20 (May 15, 1936), p. 614.

33. "New Musical in Manhattan," *Time*, September 11, 1939.

34. Edward S. Godfrey, "The New York State Program for Syphilis Control," in *Proceedings of Conference on Venereal Disease Control Work*, p. 15.

35. O. C. Wengler quoted in Poirier, *Chicago's War on Syphilis*, pp. 59, 29.

36. Rachelle Yarros, *Modern Woman and the Feminist Physician* (New York: Vanguard, 1933). For a full discussion of Yarros' role in the earlier campaign, see Alexandra M. Lord, "Naturally Clean and Wholesome: Women, Sex Education, and the United States Public Health Service, 1918–1928," *Social History of Medicine*, vol. 17, no. 3 Winter 2004), pp. 423–441.

37. "Today Is Social Hygiene Day," *Delta Star*, February 2, 1938.

38. "Local Library Joins Fight against Venereal Diseases," *Cedar Rapids Tribune*, January 14, 1938.

39. "Biggest Problem."

40. "Pupils Suffer Social Disease Rotary Told," *Middletown Times Herald*, January 19, 1937.

41. Howard M. Bell, *Youth Tell Their Story* (Washington, D.C., 1938).

42. Original italics. Benjamin C. Gruenberg, *High Schools and Sex Education* (Washington, D.C.: Public Health Service, 1940), pp. xii–xiii.

43. Ibid., p. 18.

44. "Parents' Job to Teach Sex, Says Doctor," *Hammond Times*, December 8, 1937; "Teacher Snips Evolution Text," *Hammond Times*, December 8, 1937.

45. For discussions of the contested nature of sex education programs in various different school districts, see Jeffrey Moran, *Teaching Sex: The Shaping of Adolescence in the Twentieth Century* (Cambridge, Mass.: Harvard University Press, 2000), and Janice M. Irvine, *Talk about Sex: The Battles over Sex Education in the United States* (Berkeley: University of California Press, 2002).

46. Excepts from *The Fiat Lux* (Alfred University) and *The Belfrey* (Moravian College for Women) quoted in the statement of Howard Ennes, President, Intercollegiate Association of the Middle Atlantic States, Chairman, Washington Youth Social Hygiene Council, *Hearings . . . on S. 3290*, p. 113.

47. *Gonorrhea: Its Cause, Its Spread, and Its Cure* (Washington, D.C.: Public Health Service, 1937), p. 1; *Syphilis: Its Cause, Its Spread, and Its Cure* (Washington, D.C.: Public Health Service, 1937), p. 1.

48. Robert N. Proctor, *Racial Hygiene: Medicine under the Nazis* (Cambridge, Mass.: Harvard University Press, 1988), p. 183.

49. Today these terms are associated with the rise of Nazism, but these concepts were not unique to Germany. Throughout the early twentieth century many Americans embraced the theory of eugenics, and laws in many different states reflected these concerns. Sterilization of the unfit was actually practiced in the United States during the 1920s and 1930s. See, for example, Daniel J. Kevles, *In the Name of Eugenics: Genetics and the Uses of Human Heredity* (Cambridge, Mass.: Harvard University Press, 1985), p. 111. By 1940, however, Benjamin Gruenberg and the PHS were worried that their use of the term "racial hygiene" would be misinterpreted, and they provided careful explanations of the term when discussing its relationship to sex education and venereal disease. Gruenberg, *High Schools and Sex Education*, p. xx.

50. *Gonorrhea: Its Cause, Its Spread, and Its Cure*, p. 6; *Syphilis: Its Cause, Its Spread, and Its Cure*, p. 7. The government had at different times provided soldiers and sailors with this type of advice, but this was the first time the PHS was prepared to provide such information to the general public.

51. The case was *Young Rubber v. C. I. Lee*. For a full discussion of the case and its implications, see Andrea Tone, *Devices and Desires: A History of Contraceptives in America* (New York: Hill and Wang, 2001), p. 70, and Rickie Solinger, *Pregnancy and Power: A Short History of Reproductive Politics in America* (New York: New York University Press, 2005), p. 106.

52. Mary McCarthy, *How I Grew* (New York: Harcourt, Brace, and Jovanovich, 1987), p. 77.

53. *Annual Report of the Public Health Service* (Washington, D.C.: Public Health Service, 1938), p. 133.

FOUR: Lifting the Shadow from the Land, 1941–1945

1. "Washington's High Syphilis Rate Ires Health Officials," *Wisconsin State Journal*, November 3, 1941; "Capital of Ill Health," *Time*, April 7, 1941.

2. "Civilian Aid to Social Hygiene," *The Robisonian*, February 25, 1942.

3. "North Carolina Believes VD Can Be Licked," *Northwest Arkansas Times*, June 24, 1944.

4. "Boys Meet Girls," *Time*, December 16, 1940. Even before the war began, the lack of amenities for men in training camps was evident. William O'Neill, *A Democracy at War: America's Fight at Home and Abroad* (Cambridge, Mass.: Harvard University Press, 1993), p. 89.

5. "The Doctor Tells the Story: Our Town, the Front Line of Venereal Disease Defense," *Limestone Democrat*, February 20, 1941.

6. Thomas Parran, "Public Health Also a Part of Defense Aims," *San Antonio Light*, January 12, 1941.

7. Allan M. Brandt, *No Magic Bullet: A Social History of Venereal Disease in the United States since 1880* (Oxford: Oxford University Press, 1987), p. 162. For a contemporary discussion of the book and its reception, see "State Venereal Disease Control Is Highly Praised in New Book: Vigorously Attacks Army for Alleged Lack of Interest," *Capital Times*, November 21, 1941.

8. "Postscript," *Cumberland Evening Times*, November 26, 1941; "Another Enemy to Be Fought," *Brownsville Herald*, December 13, 1941; "Venereal Disease," *Dallas Morning News*, January 4, 1942; "State Venereal Disease Control Is Highly Praised in New Book."

9. Thomas Parran, *Plain Words about Venereal Disease* (Washington, D.C.: Public Health Service, 1941), p. 34. The story may have been created by Parran to make his point, which was that testing for syphilis had increased dramatically since the PHS had launched its war on venereal disease.

10. "Civilian Aid to Social Hygiene."

11. "Syphilis among Selectees," *Delta Democrat Times*, March 20, 1941. For a more general discussion of Mississippi, Underwood, and public health in the state, see Lucie Robertson Bridgforth, "The Politics of Public Health Reform: Felix J. Underwood and the Mississippi State Board of Health, 1924–1958," *Public Historian*, vol. 6, no. 3 (Summer 1984), pp. 5–26.

12. Nicholas Lehman, *The Promised Land: The Great Black Migration and How It Changed America* (New York: Vintage Books, 1991), p. 31.

13. "Washington's High Syphilis Rate Ires Health Officials."

14. Ernest George Lion, *An Experiment in the Psychiatric Treatment of Promiscuous Girls: A Psychiatric Study under the Auspices of the Venereal Disease Division of the United States Public Health Service, the California State Department of Public Health and Department of Public Health, January 1943 to June 1944* (San Francisco: San Francisco City Clinic, 1945), pp. 27, 68.

15. "War Brings Sharp Increase in Girls' Sex Delinquencies," *Dallas Morning News*, April 7, 1943.

16. "Youngsters on the Loose," *Dallas Morning News*, July 2, 1943.

17. "High School Sex Courses Are Favored," *Nevada State Journal*, June 6, 1943.

18. "Youth Problem," *Dallas Morning News*, November 19, 1943.

19. Amy Porter, "Classroom Crisis in New York City," *Dallas Morning News*, January 10, 1943.

20. "Streets Are Patrolled for Teen-Age Children," *Dallas Morning News*, December 12, 1942.

21. "Civilian Aid to Social Hygiene."

22. "Morals Decay Traced to Home, Parents Can Control Future," *Dallas Morning News*, July 5, 1943.

23. "2,500,000 Women Will Fight to Halt Vice in Service Areas," *Dallas Morning*

News, July 16, 1942; "North Carolina Uses Mass Education to Combat VD," *Portsmouth Herald,* June 21, 1944.

24. Robert Griffith, "The Selling of America: The War Advertising Council and American Politics," *Business History Review,* vol. 57 (Autumn 1983), pp. 388–412; Maureen Honey, *Creating Rosie the Riveter: Class, Gender, and Propaganda during World War II* (Amherst: University of Massachusetts Press, 1984), pp. 31–35; "The VD Campaign," *Ada Evening News,* October 12, 1944; "Sinful, Shameful," *Time,* October 16, 1944.

25. Raymond Vonderlehr quoted in John Parascandola, *Sex, Sin, and Science: A History of Syphilis in America* (Westport, Conn.: Praeger, 2008), p. 111. For a more detailed discussion of the film, see ibid., pp. 110–112.

26. O'Neill, *Democracy at War,* p. 130.

27. Crime rates actually went down during the war. Ibid., p. 250.

28. "War Brings Sharp Increase in Girls' Sex Delinquencies." For a broader discussion of how social workers and other experts viewed this problem and its causes, see Jeffrey Moran, *Teaching Sex: The Shaping of Adolescence in the Twentieth Century* (Cambridge, Mass.: Harvard University Press, 2000), p. 121.

29. "High School Sex Courses Are Favored"; "2,500,000 Women Will Fight"; "Education Urged as Only Way to Cut Crippling Syphilis Toll," *Dallas Morning News,* March 2, 1944.

30. Thomas Snyder, ed., *120 Years of American Education: A Statistical Portrait* (Washington, D.C.: National Center for Educational Statistics, 1993), p. 18.

31. Andrew Spaull, "World War II and the Secondary School Curriculum: USA and Australia," in *Education and the Second World War: Studies in Schooling and Social Change,* ed. Roy Lowe (London: Falmer, 1992), p. 168.

32. "Venereal Ills to Be Seen in School Movies," *Dallas Morning News,* March 21, 1943; "Plans Laid to Take Drive on Venereal Ills into Public Schools," *Dallas Morning News,* February 3, 1944.

33. "U.S. Establishes Service to Aid in Sex Education," *Fresno Bee,* October 1, 1944.

34. "Education Urged as Only Way." In this instance the urging was done by the American Social Hygiene Association, but the PHS's cooperative agreement with ASHA meant that these two organizations often spoke with one voice during the war. The comment about flippancy was also made by an ASHA staff member. "U.S. Establishes Service to Aid in Sex Education."

35. "One Less Chaplain," *Time,* February 7, 1944; George W. Wickersham, *Marine Chaplain* (Bennington, Vt.: Merriam, 1998), p. 16. Robert McAfee Brown points out that the instructors at the Williamsburg school were all chaplains themselves, which may have meant that some had sympathy for Talbot's hard-line Methodism. Robert McAffee Brown, *Reflections over the Long Haul* (Louisville, Ky.: Westminster John Knox, 2005), p. 45.

36. Not all of these materials were directly produced by the government. *Corky the Killer,* for example, was a cartoon book produced by the American Social Hygiene Association in 1945. The book, which was clearly aimed at the military, received an endorsement from Surgeon General Thomas Parran, and this endorsement was splashed across the cover of the book.

37. Parascandola, *Sex, Sin, and Science,* p. 103.

38. Moran, *Teaching Sex,* p. 119.

39. Brandt, *No Magic Bullet,* p. 164.

40. *Fight Syphilis* (Public Health Service Film, 1942).

41. "The Fight on Syphilis," *Kansas City Star,* February 22, 1942.

42. Ironically, "war conditions delayed production of prints," with the result that this film could not be released during the war. *Annual Report of the Federal Security Agency* (Washington, D.C.: Public Health Service, 1945), p. 300.

43. *Fight Syphilis.*

44. Ibid.

45. "Cured by the Draft," *Time,* October 5, 1942. This latter phrase was actually the title of a chapter in Parran's book. See Parran, *Plain Words about Venereal Disease,* pp. 49–66.

46. Before 1935, treatment with Salvarsan took eighteen months. In 1935 the introduction of a continuous intravenous drip method of administering arsenical drugs radically shortened the treatment time to anywhere between ten days and six months.

47. Donna Pearce quoted in Parascandola, *Sex, Sin, and Science,* p. 120.

48. Marilyn Hegary, *Victory Girls, Khaki-wackis, and Patriotutes: The Regulation of Female Sexuality during World War II* (New York: New York University Press, 2008), p. 17.

49. *Milestones in Venereal Disease Control* (Washington, D.C.: Public Health Service, 1957), p. 7. In later years the PHS credited the rapid treatment centers with playing the central role in lowering rates of venereal disease. See *The National Venereal Disease Control Program* (Washington, D.C.: Public Health Service, 1951), p. 1.

50. Hegary, *Victory Girls, Khaki-wackis and Patriotutes,* p. 22.

51. It could be argued that with the advent of the war, young men at least would have undergone mandatory testing for syphilis.

FIVE: A False Sense of Security, 1946–1959

1. J. D. Salinger, *The Catcher in the Rye* (Boston: Little, Brown and Co., 1951), p. 120.

2. Brett Harvey, *The Fifties: A Women's Oral History* (Lincoln, Neb.: ASJA, 1993), p. 7.

3. Stephanie Coontz, *The Way We Never Were: American Families and the Nostalgia Trap* (New York: Basic Books, 1992; rpt. 2000), p. 39.

4. "Family Planning," *Time,* August 12, 1957.

5. Jeffrey Moran, *Teaching Sex: The Shaping of Adolescence in the Twentieth Century* (Cambridge, Mass.: Harvard University Press, 2000), p. 160. See also Janice Levine, *Talk about Sex: The Battle over Sex Education in the United States* (Berkeley: University of California Press, 2002), p. 18.

6. *Venereal Disease Control Seminar: Regions IX and X, Department of Health, Education, and Welfare* (Washington, D.C.: Public Health Service, 1953), p. 1.

7. "Mary Haworth's Mail: Interested Parties at Odds in Planning Girl's Future," *Dallas Morning News,* August 19, 1957.

8. "Youth Problem," *Dallas Morning News,* November 19, 1943.

9. Elaine Tyler May, *Homeward Bound: American Families in the Cold War Era* (New York: Basic Books, 1988; rpt. 1999), p. 88.

10. Beth L. Bailey, *From Front Porch to Back Seat: Courtship in Twentieth-Century America* (Baltimore: Johns Hopkins University Press, 1988), p. 42; *Women's Home Companion* (1949) quoted in ibid., p. 47.

11. Moran, *Teaching Sex,* pp. 138–153.

12. May, *Homeward Bound,* p. 121.

13. Ibid.

14. Bill Bryson, *The Life and Times of the Thunderbolt Kid: A Memoir* (New York: Broadway Books, 2006), p. 37.

15. Elizabeth Watkins points out that in the absence of aggressive action by married women, Margaret Sanger played a major role in promoting this issue during this period. Elizabeth Watkins, *On the Pill: A Social History of Oral Contraceptives, 1950–1970* (Baltimore: Johns Hopkins University Press, 1998), pp. 12–13.

16. Donald T. Critchlow, *Intended Consequences: Birth Control, Abortion, and the Federal Government in Modern America* (Oxford: Oxford University Press, 1998), pp. 15–16.

17. Gunnar Myrdal quoted in ibid., p. 34.

18. Report of the Interdepartmental Committee on Puerto Rico quoted in Linda Gordon, *The Moral Property of Women: A History of Birth Control Politics in America* (Champaign-Urbana: University of Illinois Press, 2002), p. 239.

19. Watkins, *On The Pill*, p. 19.

20. Gregory Goodwin Pincus quoted in Gordon, *Moral Property of Women*, p. 287.

21. The Catholic Church in Britain did not issue the same condemnations. "New Picture," *Time*, December 24, 1956; "The Trouble with Baby Doll," *Time*, January 14, 1957.

22. Paul Starr points to a clear element of anti-Semitism in this attack on Hollywood. Paul Starr, *The Creation of the Media: Political Origins of Modern Communications* (New York: Basic Books, 2004), p. 323.

23. Caryl Rivers, *Virgins* (New York: Pocket Books, 1984), p. 137. See also Rivers' memoir *Occasional Sins* (New York: Pocket Books, 1987).

24. Frank Sinatra quoted in Stephen J. Whitfield, *The Culture of the Cold War* (Baltimore: Johns Hopkins University Press, 1991; rpt. 1996), p. 86.

25. Frank Donough quoted in May, *Homeward Bound*, p. 126.

26. "White Girls, Negro Youths in Sex Orgies" and "Waif Center Is Shanghai Boy's Town," *Anniston Star*, October 15, 1948.

27. Nancy Gregory, "The Gay and Lesbian Movement in the United States," in *Doing Democracy: The MAP Model for Social Movements*, ed. Bill Moyer et al. (Gabriola Island, B.C.: New Society, 2001), pp. 153–164, 153.

28. "DDT Paint," *Time*, December 25, 1944.

29. My italics. Sidney Olansky quoted in Elizabeth Etheridge, *Sentinel for Health: A History of the Centers for Disease Control* (Berkeley: University of California Press, 1992), p. 88.

30. Ibid., p. 90; *Venereal Disease in Children and Youth* (Washington, D.C.: Public Health Service, 1960), p. 27.

31. *Venereal Disease Control Seminar: Region II, Federal Security Agency* (Washington, D.C.: Public Health Service, 1951), p. 29.

32. Fitzhugh Mullan, *Plagues and Politics: The Story of the United States Public Health Service* (New York: Basic Books, 1989), p. 122.

33. At this time most universities forbade hires of married couples on the grounds of nepotism. NIH, which allowed couples to be hired, attracted many leading scientists who were eager to work in an environment that allowed their spouse to find work as well.

34. The NIH had moved to the campus before the war, and its growth in many ways predated the war. However, this growth became most visible to the general public and federal employees during and immediately after the war.

35. Raymond Vondherlehr quoted in Sandra Crouse Quinn and Stephen B. Thomas,

"The National Negro Health Week, 1915–1951: A Descriptive Account," *Minority Health Today*, vol. 2, no. 3 (March–April 2001), p. 45. For a broader discussion of this program and its early demise, see Sheena M. Morrison, "Beyond the Pale: National Negro Health Week," Ph.D. diss., Columbia University, forthcoming.

36. "Parents Blamed in Sex Problems," *Holland (Michigan) Evening Sentinel*, June 15, 1949.

37. "Bring Sex out in Open, Parents Told," *Brownsville Herald*, October 19, 1948. The story was from the Associated Press.

38. *Venereal Disease Control Seminar*, p. 31.

39. "VD Meeting Set for Sunday," *Evening Capital*, March 17, 1949.

40. *The National Venereal Disease Control Program* (Washington, D.C.: Public Health Service, 1957; updated from 1951), p. 1.

41. "Family Unit Called Bulwark against Foreign Ideologies," *Chester Times*, February 21, 1950.

42. Walter Winchell, "V. (Very) D. (Dangerous)," *Port Arthur News*, November 2, 1946.

43. Weldy Bigelow, "Guest Editorial," *Standard Examiner*, June 14, 1947.

44. "Parents Blamed in Sex Problems"; "Stripe Tease," *Holland (Michigan) Evening Sentinel*, June 15, 1949.

45. *Venereal Disease Control Seminar*, p. 31.

46. "US Health Service Says Alarming Number of Teenagers Play Losing Game with VD," *Humboldt Standard*, June 7, 1956.

47. *Venereal Disease in Children and Youth* (Washington, D.C.: Public Health Service, 1960), pp. 8, 13.

SIX: Making Love, Not Babies or Disease, 1960–1980

1. *The Eradication of Syphilis: A Task Force Report to the Surgeon General Public Health Service on Syphilis Control in the United States* (Washington, D.C.: Public Health Service, 1962).

2. *Poe v. Ullman*, 367, US 497, 81, S. Ct. 1752, 6L.Ed. 2d 989 (1961) combined two actions brought in a Connecticut Superior Court. Buxton argued that the state's ban on contraceptives had prevented him from providing the best medical advice to two of his patients, both of whom had undergone dangerous and problematic pregnancies. In response to the Buxton case, the court stated that the time was not yet ripe to decide the issue. In 1965 the same issue appeared before the court. *Griswold vs. Connecticut*, 381 US 479, 85 S. Ct. 1678, 14, L.Ed. 2d 510 (1965). This time the court ruled that using contraceptives, providing advice about contraceptives, and providing contraceptives were no longer illegal.

3. *Strictly for Teenagers* (Washington, D.C.: Public Health Service, 1964), p. 4.

4. *Eradication of Syphilis*, pp. ii, 5.

5. Joseph Kershaw was the first assistant director for research and planning at the Office of Economic Opportunity, the agency that oversaw the War on Poverty. Kershaw said that when "we looked into family planning with some care . . . [we] were amazed to discover that it was probably the single most cost-effective anti-poverty measure." These concerns had led to the creation of the Office of Population Affairs. Joseph Kershaw quoted in Kristen Luker, *Dubious Conceptions: The Politics of Teenage Pregnancy* (Cambridge, Mass.: Harvard University Press, 1996), p. 59. But efforts to provide women with

contraceptive advice also reflected growing concerns regarding rising population levels. Interview of Reimart Ravenholdt conducted by Alexandra M. Lord, Seattle, Wash., February 2007. For another contemporary view on these concerns, see Phyllis Tilson Piotrow, *World Population Crisis: The United States Response* (New York: Praeger, 1973).

6. For a complete discussion of the LeClair case, see Beth Bailey, *Sex in the Heartland* (Cambridge, Mass.: Harvard University Press, 1999), pp. 200–205.

7. Throughout American history there have been several sexual revolutions. See, for example, John D'Emilio and Estelle B. Freedman, *Intimate Matters: A History of Sexuality in American History* (New York: Harper and Row, 1988), and Beth L. Bailey, *From Porch Swing to Back Seat: Courtship in Twentieth-Century America* (Baltimore: Johns Hopkins University Press, 1988).

8. For a broader discussion of shifting attitudes toward sex during this period, see David Allyn, *Make Love, Not War: The Sexual Revolution, an Unfettered History* (New York: Little, Brown and Co., 2000), and Bailey, *Sex in the Heartland.*

9. Some twenty years after the sexual revolution, Rick Moody revived memories of this period with his novel *The Ice Storm* (New York: Little, Brown and Co., 1994). The novel, and the film that followed in 1997, used the key party as a focal point for the disintegration of several marriages. For those who had come of age during or after the sexual revolution, these works created a misleading impression that this practice, while not common, was viewed as acceptable among sophisticated suburbanites.

10. See Bailey, *Sex in the Heartland,* pp. 200–205. Cohabitation among unmarried men and women remained at a low 3 percent throughout much of the 1970s. However, studies demonstrated that because many cohabitation arrangements were short-lived, the number of Americans engaging in this type of behavior was much higher than the numbers indicated. D'Emilio and Freedman, *Intimate Matters,* p. 311.

11. For a discussion of attitudes toward and depictions of the family on television, see Stephanie Coontz, *The Way We Never Were: American Families and the Nostalgia Trap* (New York: Basic Books, 1992). Judy Blume achieved widespread popularity in the 1970s for her books discussing divorce, masturbation, menarche, and sex. See, for example, Judy Blume, *It's Not the End of the World* (New York: Bantam Doubleday, 1972).

12. In opting to follow their own consciences, these same Catholics took the debate about birth control out of the public arena. Elizabeth Watkins, *On the Pill: A Social History of Oral Contraceptives* (Baltimore: Johns Hopkins University Press, 1998), pp. 40, 45–47, 62–63; Andrea Tone, *Devices and Desires: A History of Contraceptives in America* (New York: Hill and Wang, 2001), p. 241.

13. A major reorganization in 1968 reassigned many of the duties of the surgeon general to the assistant secretary of HEW. This period also witnessed attempts to eradicate the position of the surgeon general, and the post itself was left empty between 1973 and 1977. But while the surgeon general lost power during the 1960s and 1970s, the growth of HEW meant that the federal government maintained and even assumed many new powers to control public health during this period.

14. The most notable of these was probably Jesse Steinfeld, who became surgeon general in 1968. Steinfeld had entered the PHS when threatened by the draft during the Korean War; his service in the PHS sparked a lifelong interest in public health. Interview of Jesse Steinfeld conducted by Alexandra M. Lord, Pomona, Calif., September 2005.

15. "There is little question that these efforts had an impact. The decade after 1965 witnessed a sharp increase in the use of medical services by the poor. . . . Most of this in-

crease was probably due to Medicare and Medicaid." Paul Starr, *The Social Transforma-tion of American Medicine: The Rise of a Sovereign Profession and the Making of a Vast Indus-try* (New York: Basic Books, 1982), p. 373.

16. Innumerable journalists and even historians have claimed that Stewart stated that the age of infectious diseases had ended and the PHS could now "close the book" on them. Although this remark has often been cited in the literature, Dr. Stewart has said that he cannot recall whether or not he made this statement. When the statement is quoted, the sources referenced are either secondary sources that do not possess a citation or—as in the case of Laurie Garrett's book *The Coming Plague: Newly Emerging Diseases in a World out of Balance* (New York: Farrar, Strauss and Giroux, 1994)—reference a speech that Stewart gave at a conference in 1967. However, the published version of the speech does not contain the statement or anything close to it.

17. Interview Steinfeld conducted by Lord, September 2005.

18. See, for example, "Sex Education: How Much? How Soon?" *Saturday Evening Post*, June 29, 1968; "What Kids Still Don't Know about Sex: The Aware Generation Turns out to Be Surprisingly Ignorant," *Look*, July 28, 1970.

19. James Leo Herlihy and William Noble, *Blue Denim: A Play in Three Acts* (New York: Samuel French, 1959), pp. 24–25.

20. Public health experts continued to believe that illegitimate pregnancies were for the most part unwanted pregnancies. But this equation was not as simple as these experts believed. "Abortion and the Health Protections of Women," unpublished paper circu-lated with a memo from James Sasser to the Secretary's Committee on Health Protec-tion and Prevention, May 7, 1969, National Archives II (College Park, Md.), RG 235, box 1, Secretary's Committee on Health Protection and Prevention, Office of the Secre-tary, Department of Health, Education, and Welfare. See also Transcript of Proceedings from the March 15, 1969, meeting of the Secretary's Committee on Health Protection and Prevention, Office of the Secretary of the Department of Health, Education and Welfare, p. 19, National Archives II (College Park, Md.), RG 235, box 2, Secretary's Committee on Health Protection and Prevention, Office of the Secretary, Department of Health, Education, and Welfare.

21. Donald T. Critchlow, *Intended Consequences: Birth Control, Abortion, and the Federal Government in Modern America* (Oxford: Oxford University Press, 1999), p. 91.

22. Senator Joseph Tydings quoted in ibid., p. 92.

23. *A Survey of Research on Reproduction Related to Birth and Population Control* (Wash-ington, D.C.: Public Health Service of the United States Department of Health, Educa-tion and Welfare, 1973), p. 2.

24. Robert Aldrich MD and Ralph Wedgewood, "Examination of the Changes in the U.S. Which Affect the Health of Children and Youth," unpublished paper circulated at the February 27, 1968, meeting of the Secretary's Committee on Health Protection and Prevention, Office of the Secretary of the Department of Health, Education, and Wel-fare, p. 7, National Archives II (College Park, Md.), RG 235, box 2, Secretary's Commit-tee on Health Protection and Prevention, Office of the Secretary, Department of Health, Education, and Welfare.

25. Family Planning Services and Population Research Act of 1970, P.L. no. 91-572, 84 Stat. 1504 (1970), codified as amended at 42 U.S.C. §§ 300 et seq. (1991 and Supp. 2000).

26. *Annual Report for 1962 of the United States Department of Health, Education, and*

Welfare (Washington, D.C., 1962), p. 184; *Annual Report for 1965 of the United States Department of Health, Education, and Welfare* (Washington, D.C., 1965), p. 172. This focus on urban areas (along with the belief that rates of venereal disease were less common in rural areas) was typical of all federally funded sex education programs. In the early twentieth century the PHS had pitched its programs most aggressively at urban areas at the expense of rural areas, many of which were plagued by high rates of venereal disease. See Alexandra M. Lord, "Models of Masculinity," *Journal of the History of Medicine and Allied Sciences*, vol. 58, no. 2 (April 2003), pp. 123–153. Similarly, in the late twentieth century, AIDS quickly reached rural communities even as many Americans continued to view the disease as an "urban" problem. For one of the most revealing discussions of AIDS in rural communities, see Abraham Verghese, *My Own Country: A Doctor's Story* (New York: Vintage, 1995). The book was ultimately made into a film.

27. Transcript of Proceedings from the November 21, 1969, meeting of the Secretary's Committee on Health Protection and Prevention, Office of the Secretary of the Department of Health, Education, and Welfare, pp. 6, 8, National Archives II (College Park, Md.), RG 235, box 2, Secretary's Committee on Health Protection and Prevention, Office of the Secretary, Department of Health, Education, and Welfare.

28. Letter from Richard Prindle, Assistant Surgeon General (PHS) to Theodore Ingalls MD, dated May 27, 1969, National Archives II (College Park, Md.), RG 235, box 1, Secretary's Committee on Health Protection and Prevention, Office of the Secretary, Department of Health, Education, and Welfare.

29. Rickie Solinger, *Abortion Wars: A Half Century of Struggle, 1950–2000* (Berkeley: University of California Press, 1998) p. 17.

30. Ibid.

31. Transcript of Proceedings from the March 15, 1969, meeting of the of the Secretary's Committee on Health Protection and Prevention, p. 33.

32. Transcript of Proceedings from the November 21, 1969, meeting of the Secretary's Committee on Health Protection and Prevention, p. 14.

33. Letter from Arthur S. Fleming to Robert Finch, Secretary of the Department of Health, Education and Welfare, March 28, 1969, p. 5, National Archives II (College Park, Md.), RG 235, box 2, Secretary's Committee on Health Protection and Prevention, Office of the Secretary, Department of Health, Education, and Welfare.

34. Transcript of Proceedings from the November 21, 1969, meeting of the Secretary's Committee on Health Protection and Prevention, p. 82.

35. Unpublished paper circulated at the February 27, 1968, meeting of the Secretary's Committee on Health Protection and Prevention, Office of the Secretary of the Department of Health, Education, and Welfare, pp. 15–16.

36. Wilbur Cohen, "Health in America: The Role of the Federal Government in Bringing High Quality Health Care to All the American People," unpublished report presented to Richard M. Nixon, March 4, 1968, p. 6, National Archives II (College Park, Md.), RG 235, box 2, Secretary's Committee on Health Protection and Prevention, Office of the Secretary, Department of Health, Education, and Welfare.

37. *Strictly for Teenagers* (Washington, D.C.: Public Health Service, 1964), p. 8.

38. This presents a fascinating contrast to shows that aired in the 1990s and 2000s. On shows such as *Beverly Hills 90210* and *The OC*, the teens who opt not to have sex are the outliers. Moreover, the shows' main characters *do* engage in sex; pregnancy scares notwithstanding, the actions of these teens do not result in pregnancy or disease.

39. During the 1960s the writers for two television shows, *Mr. Novak* and *Dr. Kildare*, had created episodes in which a teenager contracted venereal disease. However, NBC ultimately refused to air the shows. Allan Brandt, *A Social History of Venereal Disease in the United States since 1880* (New York: Oxford University Press, 1986), p. 176.

40. *Teenage Pregnancy: Everyone's Problem* (Washington, D.C.: Public Health Service, 1977), pp. 3–5.

41. Medicaid reimbursements for contraceptive services were also set substantially higher than that provided for other Medicaid services: 90 percent of the cost of contraceptive services was reimbursed as compared with 50–80 percent of other services provided by Medicaid. Kristen Luker, *Dubious Conceptions: The Politics of Teenage Pregnancy* (Cambridge, Mass.: Harvard University Press, 1996), p. 59. For a discussion of inflation and its impact on these programs, see Transcript of Proceedings from the November 21, 1969, meeting of the Secretary's Committee on Health Protection and Prevention, p. 89.

42. Transcript of Proceedings from the November 21, 1969, meeting of the Secretary's Committee on Health Protection and Prevention, p. 89.

43. Mailing Sent to the Secretary's Committee on Health Protection and Prevention, November 21, 1969, National Archives II (College Park, Md.), RG 235, box 2, Secretary's Committee on Health Protection and Prevention, Office of the Secretary, Department of Health, Education, and Welfare.

44. Allan Brandt, *No Magic Bullet: A Social History of Venereal Disease in the United States since 1880* (New York: Oxford University Press, 1986), p. 178.

45. Transcript of Proceedings from the November 21, 1969, meeting of the Secretary's Committee on Health Protection and Prevention, p. 19.

46. Unpublished paper circulated at the February 27, 1968, meeting of the Secretary's Committee on Health Protection and Prevention, p. 10.

SEVEN: Telling It Like It Is, 1981–1988

1. C. Everett Koop, "The Early Days of AIDS as I Remember Them," *AIDS and the Public Debate: Historical and Contemporary Perspectives*, ed. Caroline Hannaway, Victoria Harden, and John Parascandola (Amsterdam: IOS Press, 1995), p. 9.

2. Interview of Anthony Fauci conducted by Victoria Harden, Bethesda, Md., June 29, 1993.

3. Senator Edward Kennedy, Congressional Record (Senate), November 16, 1981, §13413.

4. David W. Fisher, "The Job Grew in the Man," *Hospital Practice*, March 15, 1989, p. 9.

5. Kennedy, Congressional Record (Senate), November 16, 1981, §13413.

6. Interview of C. Everett Koop conducted by Fitzhugh Mullan, Bethesda, Md., February 6, 1989.

7. This fame was fleeting. Although Koop would continue to be lampooned and featured on shows such as *The Simpsons* throughout the 1990s and into the first decade of the twenty-first century, many Americans born after the 1980s are often unfamiliar with him.

8. Nadine Brozan, "Fathers and Sons Talk about Growing Up," *New York Times*, July 14, 1981.

9. Americans have always found information about sex in a variety of places, and this information has always varied in terms of accuracy and biases. In the 1970s and 1980s, the sheer number of sources that provided such information skyrocketed.

10. For a full discussion of Howe and the battle for sex education in the 1970s, see William Martin, *With God on Our Side: The Rise of the Religious Right* (New York: Broadway Books, 1996), pp. 100–116.

11. Jerry Falwell quoted in ibid., p. 204.

12. Ibid., p. 208.

13. Before his nomination Koop served on the boards of three different Right-to-Life organizations, and he played a major part in one of the movement's most widely released films attacking the legalization of abortion.

14. Eva Hoffman and Margot Slade, "A Policy Switch in Sex Education?" *New York Times*, February 22, 1981. Mecklenburg's appointment did not mean that she became neutral or broke ties with the pro-life movement. See, for example, Msgr. Noel C. Burtenshaw, "Marjorie Mecklenburg Sees White House Pro-Life Support," *Georgia Bulletin: The Newspaper of the Catholic Archdiocese of Atlanta*, February 10, 1983.

15. "Voices from across the Nation on Teenage Pregnancy," *USA Today*, October 14, 1987. The overwhelming majority of Americans agreed on the need for good sex education, and for the majority, "good" sex education meant programs and materials that provided people with comprehensive information. See, for example, Jeffrey Moran, *Teaching Sex: The Shaping of Adolescence in the Twentieth Century* (Cambridge, Mass.: Harvard University Press, 2002), and Janice Levine, *Talk about Sex: The Battle over Sex Education in the United States* (Berkeley: University of California Press, 2002).

16. Carter cut funding for population control programs. Interview of Reimart Ravenholt conducted by Alexandra M. Lord, Seattle, Wash., February 19, 2007.

17. C. Everett Koop, *Koop: The Memoirs of America's Family Doctor* (New York: Random House, 1981), p. 87.

18. "Koop for Surgeon General," *Christianity Today*, June 26, 1982.

19. Deirdre Wulf, "A Problem Peculiar to the USA," *USA Today*, October 14, 1987, p. 12A.

20. Interview of Leonard Bachman conducted by Alexandra M. Lord, Washington, D.C., January 2005.

21. Not everyone was a fan of Koop's visibility. See, for example, "Full Dress for the AIDS War," *Boston Globe*, April 27, 1989.

22. "A Doctor Prescribes a Hard Truth," *Time*, April 24, 1989, p. 82.

23. Jim Shahin, "Flying the Koop," *American Way Magazine*, June 15, 1989, p. 62.

24. "Six More Sexy Guys and Why We Like 'Em," *USA Weekend*, January 27–29, 1989, p. 5.

25. *Koop*, p. 26.

26. *Surgeon General's Report on Acquired Immune Deficiency Syndrome* (Washington, D.C.: Public Health Service, 1986), p. 26.

27. Ibid., p. 21.

28. Parran, for example, had found it preferable to allow people to claim that they had contracted venereal disease from a shared drinking cup or towel, provided that this enabled the sufferer to feel comfortable about publicly admitting that he or she had venereal disease.

29. *Koop*, p. 214.

30. *Surgeon General's Report on Acquired Immune Deficiency Syndrome*, p. 4.

31. *Koop*, p. 223.

32. "An Interview with C. Everett Koop: Priorities of the Surgeon General," *Nursing Economics*, vol. 6, no. 3 (May–June, 1988), p. 108.

33. *The Washingtonian*, June 1987, p. 113.

34. Julia Reed, "The Hot New Politics of AIDS," *US News and World Report*, March 30, 1987.

35. Deborah Mesce, "Koop Quitting as Surgeon General: Doctor Made Mark with Fight against AIDS and Smoking," *Los Angeles Herald Examiner*, May 5, 1989, p. A7.

36. Marlene Cimon, "Koop to Quit Surgeon General Post," *Los Angeles Times*, May 5, 1989.

37. Sandra Dunne, "Citizen Koop: The Report on the Surgeon General," *Washington Post Magazine*, November 15, 1987, p. 26.

38. Cynthia Tucker, "Koop's AIDS Report Based on Reason," *Atlanta Journal-Constitution*, October 27, 1986, p. 12.

39. *Koop*, p. 226.

40. Address by C. Everett Koop, Surgeon General of the U.S. Public Health Service, U.S. Department of Health and Human Services, Presented at Cardozo High School, Washington, D.C., February 25, 1988, Koop file, Office of the Public Health Service Historian Archives, Rockville, Md.

41. Marc Fisher, "Surgeon General Minces No Words on AIDS; Koop's Lecture at Cardozo Aims at Misinformation," *Washington Post*, February 26, 1988.

42. "A Non-Response to AIDS," *Boston Globe*, January 28, 1988, p. 22.

43. Jeffrey Zaslow, "Huge Mailing Takes AIDS Battle into Every Home," *Chicago Sun-Tribune*, July 30, 1989; interview of Leonard Bachman conducted by Alexandra M. Lord, Washington, D.C., January 2004.

44. Zaslow, "Huge Mailing Takes AIDS Battle into Every Home."

45. Sandra Broodman and Philip J. Hilts, "Plan Issued for AIDS Education: Federal Report Stresses Abstinence and Monogamy," *Washington Post*, March 17, 1987; Reed, "Hot New Politics of AIDS."

46. *Understanding AIDS* (Washington, D.C.: Public Health Service, 1988), p. 1.

47. Lewis Cope, "Straight Talk about AIDS Should Reach Every Mailbox," *Minneapolis Star-Tribune*, May 5, 1988, p. 11B.

48. "The AIDS Mailing Saga," *Boston Globe*, May 9, 1988, p. 18.

49. Zaslow, "Huge Mailing Takes AIDS Battle into Every Home."

50. Judie Brown, "This AIDS Pamphlet Fails to Face Facts," *USA Today*, June 8, 1988.

51. "AIDS Book Spells out Facts, Fiction," *USA Today*, May 5, 1988.

52. Zaslow, "Huge Mailing Takes AIDS Battle into Every Home."

EIGHT: Abstinence Makes the Heart Grow Fonder, 1989–2008

1. Monica Davey, "Palin's Daughter's Pregnancy Interrupts G.O.P. Script," *New York Times*, September 1, 2008.

2. Sara Rimer, "TV's Perfect Girl Is Pregnant, Real Families Say 'Let's Talk,'" *New*

York Times, December 21, 2007, p. A25. Rimer's story was picked up and run in other papers including the *Denver Post,* the *Santa Rosa Press Democrat,* and the *Chicago Tribune.*

3. Monthly Report of the Rapides Station Community Ministries of Louisiana (1999) quoted in *American Civil Liberties Union v. Governor M. J. Foster and Dan Richey, United States District Court for the Eastern District of Louisiana,* p. 4. For a discussion of the case itself, see Ceci Connolly, "ACLU Sues Louisiana over Abstinence Teaching," *Washington Post,* May 9, 2002, p. A29. The story was also discussed by nationally syndicated columnists. See, for example, Ellen Goodman, "The Gospel of Abstinence," *Boston Globe,* June 23, 2002.

4. Richard Owen, "Pregnant Mary Embarrasses the Pope," *The Times* (London), November 24, 2006.

5. See, for example, Ruth Marcus, "The Real Lessons of Jamie Lynn Spears' Pregnancy," *Los Angeles Times,* December 28, 2007; Kristen Kennedy, "Let's Talk about Sex: With Jamie Lynn Spears' Pregnancy Now Is a Good Time to Have the 'Big Talk' with Your Teen," *MSN.com;* David Crary, "In Movies and Real Life Pregnant Teens Spark Debate," *Charleston Gazette,* December 21, 2007; Monica Hess, "The Other Spears Does the Bump: Britney's Little Sister No Longer the, Uh, Role Model," *Washington Post,* December 20, 2007; Ruth Marcus, "The Lesson of Bristol Palin," *Washington Post,* September 2, 2008; Linda Hirshman, "Do as We Do," *Slate.com,* September 2, 2008.

6. Opponents of birth control had a long history of linking patriotism with opposition to birth control. Strong ties between opponents of birth control and adherents of organizations such as the John Birch Society also meant that sex education was linked with communism and "anti-Americanism" in general. See William Martin, *With God on Our Side: The Rise of the Religious Right in America* (New York: Broadway Books, 1996), p. 119; Jeffrey Moran, *Teaching Sex: The Shaping of Adolescence in the Twentieth Century* (Cambridge, Mass.: Harvard University Press, 2000), pp. 179–183.

7. Sally Squires, "Front Runner for Surgeon General," *Washington Post,* October 24, 1989. Novello was forty-five when she was appointed. She herself later admitted that her relative youth had been a handicap in the job, as she was concerned about her future career. Interview of Antonia Novello conducted by Alexandra M. Lord, Albany, N.Y., December 2005.

8. Michael Spector, "What's America Doing in Bed? We Need a National Sex Survey to Fight AIDS Effectively So Why Is Congress Ducking It?" *Washington Post,* February 25, 1990; Nancy Gibbs, "Teens: The Rising Risk of AIDS," *Time,* September 2, 1991.

9. Moran, *Teaching Sex,* p. 208.

10. For a full discussion of the creation of the Adolescent Family Life Act, the lawsuit that ensued, and the impact of the program on sex education in general, see Janice M. Irvine, *Talk about Sex: The Battles over Sex Education in the United States* (Berkeley: University of California Press, 2002), pp. 90–106, and Rebekkah Saul, "Whatever Happened to the Adolescent Family Life Act?" *Guttmacher Report on Public Policy,* vol. 1, no. 2 (April 1998).

11. Cynthia Dailard, "Sex Education, Parents, Politics and Teens," *Guttmacher Report on Public Policy,* vol. 4, no. 1 (February 2001).

12. Tracy Thompson, "House Panel Asserts Delay on AIDS Report Is Political," *Washington Post,* October 9, 1992.

13. *Surgeon General's Report to the American People on HIV Infection and AIDS* (Washington, D.C.: Department of Health and Human Services, 1992), p. 22.

14. Ibid., pp. 14, 6.

15. Megan Rosenfeld, "Bush's Unlikely Family Man: He's Unmarried, Abstinent and in Charge of Contraception," *Washington Post*, August 5, 1992. Archer would go on to serve other members of the Bush family. In 1997 then-governor of Texas George W. Bush appointed Archer as his commissioner of health. In 2000, while running for president, Bush was forced to put Archer on leave. That year Archer publicly "minimized the importance of health insurance and said the Hispanic population lacked the belief 'that getting pregnant is a bad thing.' " "Official Who Embarrassed Bush Is Removed," *New York Times*, October 20, 2000. Archer formally resigned three days after the article in the *New York Times* appeared, and his boss, George W. Bush, went on to win the presidency later that year.

16. Susan Tifft, "Better Safe Than Sorry?" *Time*, January 21, 1991; "Majority of US Adults Favor Distribution of Condoms in Public Schools, Poll Finds," *Daily Women's Health Policy Report (Kaiser Family Foundation)*, November 2, 2007; Nancy Gibbs, "Teens: The Rising Risk of AIDS," *Time*, September 2, 1991.

17. "Elders: You Can't Get Tired and Sit Down," *Journal of NIH Research*, vol. 5, no. 9, (September 1993), p. 40; Joyce Price, "Senate Panel Mum on Eve of Elders Hearing," *Washington Times*, July 23, 1993, p. A3; John Schwartz, "Elders Ends Silence before Senate Panel," *Washington Post*, July 24, 1993. Elders also pointed out that her decision not to make a public announcement regarding condoms' flaws had been shaped by her understanding of public health. " 'As public health decision, you try to do the greatest good' for the greatest number of people," Elders told the Senate. Ironically, time may have proved Elders' decision to be correct. Throughout the 1990s and well into the twenty-first century, many abstinence-only programs have focused on possible flaws in condoms. When students in these abstinence-only programs engage in sex—and they do engage in sex—they are less likely to use condoms than their peers who attend comprehensive sex education programs. Public health experts believe that these teens' reluctance to use condoms stems from their belief that condoms are ineffective.

18. Paul Henrickson, "Elders' Prescription for Battle: Outspoken and Upfront: Here's Clinton's Pick for Surgeon General," *Washington Post*, February 16, 1993; Floyd Brown, "Life and Death in Arkansas: Dr. Joycelyn Elders Does Not Hide Her Contempt for Those Who Prefer Life to 'Quality of Life,' " *National Review*, April 26, 1993.

19. Price, "Senate Panel Mum on Eve of Elders Hearing"; Laurie Goodstein, "Nominee Draws Attacks, Support from Religious Groups," *Washington Post*, July 24, 1993, p. A8; Thomas L. Friedman, "Battle Likely over Nominee for Surgeon General," *New York Times*, July 10, 1993, p. 8; Jesse Jackson, "Elders Is a Nominee Worth a Fight," *Los Angeles Times*, July 26, 1993; "Dr. Joycelyn Elders an Excellent Choice for Surgeon General," *Philadelphia Inquirer*, July 15, 1993; Lynn Rosellini, "The Prescriptions of Dr. Yes," *US News and World Report*, July 26, 1993; Cal Thomas and Suzanne Fields, "Listening to Elders and Saying No," *Washington Times*, July 15, 1993.

20. Helen Dewar, "Elders Is Confirmed as Surgeon General: GOP Conservatives Fail to Derail Nomination," *Washington Post*, September 8, 1993, p. A4.

21. M. Joycelyn Elders, "Saving Our Children: Acceptance Speech for the Alvin C. Eurich Education Achievement Award," June 23, 1993 (New York: Academy for Educational Development, 1993), p. 8.

22. "An Interview with the Surgeon General," *Commissioned Corps Bulletin*, vol. 7, no. 3 (November 1993), p. 2.

23. Multiple studies sponsored by diverse groups have indicated that teens' decisions to have sex and/or become pregnant stem from diverse factors. For the best and most comprehensive discussion of this, see Kristen Lucker, *Dubious Conceptions: The Politics of Teenage Pregnancy* (Cambridge, Mass.: Harvard University Press, 1996). For a more recent discussion, see, for example, E. M. Saewyc, L. L. Magee, and S. E. Pettingell, "Teenage Pregnancy and Associated Risk Behaviors among Sexually Abused Adolescents," *Perspectives on Sexual and Reproductive Health*, vol. 36, no. 3 (May–June 2004), pp. 98–105, and J. Manlove, "The Influence of High School Dropout and School Disengagement on the Risk of School-Age Pregnancy," *Journal of Research on Adolescence*, vol. 8, no. 2 (1998), pp. 187–220. When speaking to public health experts, Elders acknowledged the complexity of this issue. See Joycelyn Elders, "The Future of US Public Health," *JAMA*, vol. 269, no. 17 (May 5, 1993), p. 2293.

24. Claudia Dreifus, "Joycelyn Elders," *New York Times Magazine*, January 30, 1994; Rosellini, "Prescriptions of Dr. Yes."

25. "Surgeon General Urges Sex Ed for Students in Grades K–12," *Jet*, December 20, 1993; "Quotes by and about Joycelyn Elders," [Knight-Ridder] *Tribune*, December 9, 1994; Philip J. Hilts, "Blunt Style Proves Asset for Elders," *Journal Record*, September 15, 1993.

26. Vanessa Gallman, "The Surgeon General's Opinions Are Bitter Pills to Many," *Philadelphia Inquirer*, September 15, 1994; Robert Novak, "Elders a Malaise Clinton Can't Cure," *Chicago Sun-Times*, June 23, 1994.

27. Philip J. Hilts, "Blunt Style Proves Asset for Elders."

28. "Republicans Call for Elders' Ouster: Surgeon General's Criticisms of Religious Right Leads to Clash," *Washington Post*, June 26, 1994. The attacks were marshaled in part by those already planning a run against Clinton in 1996. When commenting on the attacks against Elders, Clinton angrily "said he was tired of being pounded by the Christian Right," and he vowed to be more aggressive in fighting off the attacks in the future. Escalating accusations leveled against Clinton for his own sexual behavior ultimately made it impossible for him to respond to these attacks. Calls for Elders to be dismissed also stemmed from her public comments on drugs. "Don't Ask Dr. Elders," *The Nation*, December 27, 1993. Elders' credibility on this issue was tarnished when her son was arrested for selling cocaine.

29. Both Clinton and Gingrich were ultimately forced to admit that while married they had engaged in sexual relationships with younger women who were not their wives.

30. Martin, *With God on Our Side*, pp. 171–172.

31. "Controversial Joycelyn Elders," *The Record*, January 4, 1995; Juliet Wittman, "Joycelyn Elders Silenced by Newt's Values," Knight-Ridder / Tribune News Service, December 22, 1994; Cameron Bryon "What Do You Think of Clinton's Dismissal of Elders?" *Boston Globe*, December 14, 1994; "Sad to See Elders Go," *Washington Post*, December 29, 1994; William Egyir, "Protests Greet Clinton's Dismissal of Elders as Surgeon General," *Amsterdam News*, December 17, 1994; "Surgeon General Fought Hard for Youth," *New York Times*, December 14, 1994.

32. Laurie Goodstein, "Southern Baptists Urge Opposition to Foster, Positions on Abortion, Sex Education Criticized," *Washington Post*, February 23, 1995; Reginold

Bundy, "A Different Breed from Elders," *Tri-State Defender,* February 15, 1995; "Black Churches Divided over Foster's Nomination," *Christian Century,* May 17, 1995.

33. "David Satcher Faces High-Profile Challenges as 'America's Doctor,'" *Virginian-Pilot,* February 11, 1998; Helen Dewar, "Senate Confirms David Satcher as Surgeon General," *Washington Post,* February 11, 1998. The *Washington Post* speculated that Ashcroft's opposition to Satcher stemmed in large part from Ashcroft's plans to run for president in 2000.

34. Chris Bull, "The Calm after the Storm," *The Advocate,* May 25, 1999; Sheryl Gay Stolberg, "Scientist at Work: Satcher, Tiptoeing through the Minefields of Health Policy," *New York Times,* April 21, 1998.

35. Stolberg, "Scientist at Work"; Bull, "Calm after the Storm."

36. David Satcher, "A Letter from the Surgeon General," in *The Surgeon General's Call to Action to Promote Sexual Health and Responsible Sexual Behavior* (Washington, D.C.: Department of Health and Human Services, 21), pp. 1–2.

37. Michael Castleman, "A Call to Yawns," *Salon,* July 29, 2001; Deborah Mathis, "Sex and the Surgeon General," *Seattle Post-Intelligencer,* July 6, 2001.

38. Tommy Thompson and Ari Fleischer quoted in *Talk of the Nation with Juan Williams,* NPR Radio, July 3, 2001.

39. Even well-intentioned parents fell down on the job. A study released in the same period as Satcher's Call to Action indicated that while many mothers believed that they had provided their daughters with sex education, their daughters disagreed. "Has There Been a Talk about Sex? Teenagers and Their Mothers Often Disagree," *International Family Planning Perspectives,* vol. 32, no. 4 (July–August 2000).

40. *Impact of Four Title V, Section 51 Abstinence Education Programs,* Mathematica Policy Research, submitted in April 2007, contract no. HHS 100-98-0010, Department of Health and Human Services, p. xiv. The full report is available at www.mathematica-mpr.com/publications/pdfs/impactabstinence.pdf.

41. Representative Lois Capps quoted in Susan Rose, "Going Too Far? Sex, Sin, and Social Policy," *Social Forces,* December 1, 2005. The impact of these scare tactics was demonstrated by a survey conducted by the Kaiser Family Foundation in 2000. Almost one in five students surveyed said that their teachers presented sex as "something to fear and avoid." Irvine, *Talk about Sex,* p. 121.

42. *The Content of Federally Funded Abstinence-Only Education Programs Prepared for Henry Waxman* (Washington, D.C.: House of Representatives Committee on Government Reform, Minority Staff Special Investigations Division, December 2004), pp. I, 22, 17–18.

43. Ceci Connolly, "Some Abstinence Programs Mislead Teens, Report Finds," *Washington Post,* December 2, 2004.

44. After his resignation Carmona publicly testified to his conviction that he had been stifled by the Bush administration. Carmona stated that in regard to sex education, the Bush administration "did not want to hear the science but wanted to just preach abstinence which I felt was incorrect." "Ex–Surgeon General Says Theology Not Science Drives Agenda under Bush," *Church and State,* September 1, 2007; Gardiner Harris, "Surgeon General Sees 4 Year Term as Compromised," *New York Times,* July 11, 2007.

45. Adolescents who received comprehensive sex education had a lower risk of pregnancy than adolescents who received abstinence-only or no sex education. P. K. Kohler,

L. E. Manhart, and W. E. Lafferty, "Abstinence-Only and Comprehensive Sex Education and the Initiation of Sexual Activity and Teen Pregnancy," *Journal of Adolescent Health*, vol. 42, no. 4 (April 2008), pp. 344–351. Findings of another study indicated that adolescents who received comprehensive sex education and those who received abstinence-only education did not engage in different patterns of sexual activity. C. Trenholm et al., "Impacts of Abstinence Education on Teen Sexual Activity, Risk of Pregnancy, and Risk of Sexually Transmitted Diseases," *Journal of Policy Analysis and Management*, vol. 27, no. 2 (Spring 2008), pp. 255–276. See also Margaret Talbot, "Red Sex, Blue Sex," *The New Yorker*, November 3, 2008, pp. 64–69.

46. "Ex-Surgeon General Says Theology Not Science Drives Agenda under Bush"; Harris, "Surgeon General Sees 4 Year Term as Compromised."

47. Two websites were specifically cited as problematic. In 2003 a website sponsored by the CDC was withdrawn and rewritten to imply a link between abortion and breast cancer. No evidence for such a link exists. The individual who made the claim on the CDC website later received a contract to write a website on sex education for parents and teenagers. The latter website was also discovered to be deeply problematic. Several statements, including one that claims that teenagers engage in sex because they have access to condoms, have no basis in fact. "US Is Asked to Close Site on Sex Issues," *New York Times*, April 3, 2005; Phil Wilson, "It Doesn't Matter Whether Bush Loves Us," *New York Beacon*, October 12, 2005; Jennifer Block, "Sex, Lies and Duct Tape," *Conscience*, March 22, 2003; Ceci Connolly, "Panel Finds Misinformation in White House Web Site on Teenagers: Negative Messages about Gays, Single Parents Criticized as Well as Lack of Information on Alcohol," *Washington Post*, July 14, 2005; "McManus Feeds at Public Trough," *State Church Bulletin*, March 1, 2005; Marc Kaufman, "Sex Ed Group Faces New Review, Government Plans a Third Look at Advocates for Youth," *Washington Post*, August 16, 2003; "Bush Policies Hurt AIDS Prevention, Groups Say, Administration Accused of Disinformation on Condom Use, Harassment, Audits of Education Programs," *Washington Post*, October 1, 2003; Christopher Healy, "No Sex Please or We'll Audit You," *Salon*, October 28, 2003.

48. The promotion of religion in abstinence-only programs dates back to Reagan, and it continued to be a problem under presidents George H. W. Bush and Bill Clinton. Under President George W. Bush, there may have been an escalation in this practice. See, for example, Jonathan Saltzman, "Abstinence Funds Are Suspended, US Halts Support after ACLU Suit," *Boston Globe*, August 24, 2005, and "God Says Wait," *Pittsburgh City Paper*, February 9, 2005.

49. Larry Rohter, "Ad on Sex Education Distorts Obama Policy," *New York Times*, September 1, 2008. See also "Off-Base on Sex Education," *FactCheck.org*, September 1, 2008, updated September 18, 2008, www.factcheck.org/elections-2008/off_base_on_sex _ed.html.

50. See *The Parents' Part* (Washington, D.C.: Public Health Service, 1918). The pamphlet called upon parents, ministers, and teachers to provide their children with age-appropriate sex education when the child was four or five.

51. "Obama Says Palin's Family Off-Limits" September 2, 2008, www.cnn.com/ 2008/POLITICS/09/01/obama.palin/index.html.

52. "Group Protests outside Obama's Local Campaign Office," September 29, 2008, www.kktv.com/home/headlines/29994109.html#comments.

Epilogue

1. "Dear Beth," *Boston Globe*, April 2, 1987.
2. Although adolescents and young adults have often engaged in premarital sex, pressure to marry has kept illegitimacy rates low. However, when historians correlate birth dates and marriage dates, it is clear that significant percentages of American brides were pregnant at marriage. In the Chesapeake Bay area during the seventeenth century, for example, 30 percent of brides were already pregnant when they married. Low levels of nutrition (which can impact fertility rates) probably kept the number of early births at a low level. John D'Emilio and Estelle B. Freedman, *Intimate Matters: A History of Sexuality in America* (Chicago: University of Chicago Press, 1998), pp. 16–27.
3. Sharon Lerner, "The Sex Ed Divide," *American Prospect*, vol. 12, no. 17 (September 24–October 8, 2001). Research for this article was supported by a grant from the Kaiser Family Foundation and the National Press Foundation.
4. There is evidence that the Bush administration attempted to suppress these findings. John Santelli, "Abstinence-Only Education: Politics, Science, and Ethics," *Social Research*, September 22, 2006.
5. Mark Sherman, "Bush Pushes Abstinence Education," *Charleston Gazette*, November 26, 2004. Throughout his tenure in the Bush administration, Horn was an extremely controversial figure. "Former HHS Official Wade F. Horn Funded Group That He Fathered," *Church and State*, May 1, 2007.
6. "Abstinence-Only Fails to Protect Teens," *Albuquerque State Journal*, December 19, 2007.

INDEX

Page numbers in *italics* indicate illustrations.